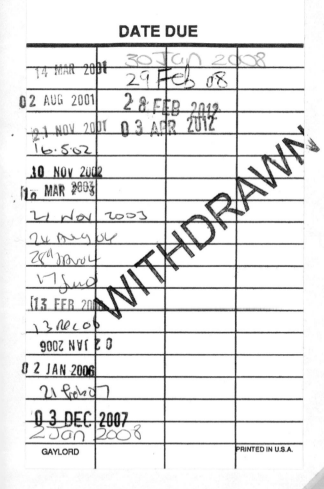

The Mental Health Nurse
Views of Practice and Education

Also available from Blackwell Science

Mental Health Law for Nurses
Bridgit C. Dimond and Frances H. Barker
0 632 03989 2

Journal of Psychiatric and Mental Health Nursing
Editor: Bill Lemmer
ISSN 1351-0126

Journal of Psychiatric and Mental Health Nursing is a peer-reviewed journal that publishes original contributions which integrate the knowledge and practice of psychiatric and mental health nursing.

It provides an international forum for all professionals in this field and is dedicated to the development of knowledge through description and evaluation.

Journal of Psychiatric and Mental Health Nursing:

- emphasises the importance of the consumer as an active collaborator
- acknowledges the experience of care and caring
- emphasises human values, providing a forum that widens access to support, information and expertise

Journal of Psychiatric and Mental Health Nursing is published bimonthly.

The Mental Health Nurse

Views of Practice and Education

Edited by

Stephen Tilley

Blackwell
Science

© 1997 by
Blackwell Science Ltd
Editorial Offices:
Osney Mead, Oxford OX2 0EL
25 John Street, London WC1N 2BL
23 Ainslie Place, Edinburgh EH3 6AJ
350 Main Street, Malden
  MA 02148 5018, USA
54 University Street, Carlton
  Victoria 3053, Australia

Other Editorial Offices:

Blackwell Wissenschafts-Verlag GmbH
Kurfürstendamm 57
10707 Berlin, Germany

Blackwell Science KK
MG Kodenmacho Building
7–10 Kodenmacho Nihombashi
Chuo-ku, Tokyo 104, Japan

First published 1997

Set in 10/12 Palatino
by DP Photosetting, Aylesbury, Bucks
Printed and bound in Great Britain by
Hartnolls Ltd, Bodmin, Cornwall

The Blackwell Science logo is a
trade mark of Blackwell Science Ltd,
registered at the United Kingdom
Trade Marks Registry

DISTRIBUTORS
Marston Book Services Ltd
PO Box 269
Abingdon
Oxon OX14 4YN
(*Orders:* Tel: 01235 465500
        Fax: 01235 465555)

USA
Blackwell Science, Inc.
Commerce Place
350 Main Street
Malden, MA 02148 5018
(*Orders:* Tel: 800 759 6102
                617 388 8250
         Fax: 617 388 8255)

Canada
Copp Clark Professional
200 Adelaide Street West, 3rd Floor
Toronto, Ontario M5H 1W7
(*Orders:* Tel: 416 597 1616
                800 815 9417
         Fax: 416 597 1617)

Australia
Blackwell Science Pty Ltd
54 University Street
Carlton, Victoria 3053
(*Orders:* Tel: 03 9347 0300
         Fax: 03 9347 5001)

A catalogue record for this title
is available from the British Library

ISBN 0-632-03999-X

Contents

List of Contributors

Annie Altschul   CBE, BA, MSc, RGN, RMN, RNT, FRCN
Emeritus Professor of Nursing Studies, The University of Edinburgh

Phil Barker   PhD, RN
Professor of Psychiatric Nursing Practice, Department of Neuroscience and Psychiatry, University of Newcastle-upon-Tyne

Ruth M. Gallop   BScN, MScN, PhD, RN
Associate Professor, Faculty of Nursing, University of Toronto, Canada

David Glenister   BSc, RMN, MSc, PGCEA
Health Studies Fellow, Practice Development Unit, Health and Social Services Institute, University of Essex, Colchester

Tessa Parkes   BSc (Hons), RMN
Postgraduate Student, The Tizard Centre, University of Kent at Canterbury

Linda C. Pollock   BSc, RGN, Dist Nursing Cert, RMN, Diploma in Nursing (Edin), PhD, MBA
Nursing Director and Community General Manager, Edinburgh Healthcare NHS Trust

Susan Ritter   MA, RGN, RMN
Lecturer in Psychiatric Nursing, Institute of Psychiatry, University of London

Desmond Ryan   MA, DipSocAdmin, DPhil
Director, Health Care Education Research, School of Nursing and Midwifery, University of Dundee

Duncan Tennant   RMN, RGN, MSc
Clinical Nurse Specialist, Mental Health, West Lothian NHS Trust

Stephen Tilley   BA, PhD, RMN
Lecturer, Department of Nursing Studies, The University of Edinburgh

Christine Walsh   MA (Applied) in Social Science Research, RPN, RGON
Lecturer, Victoria University, Wellington, New Zealand

Roger Watson   BSc, PhD, RGN, CBiol, MIBiol
Senior Lecturer, Department of Nursing Studies, The University of Edinburgh

Irene Whitehill   BSc, PhD
Freelance Trainer and Consultant (Mental Health), Northumberland

Introduction

Stephen Tilley

The aim of the book

Anyone thinking about becoming a mental health nurse may want to know 'What is it I might become? By what means would I become a nurse?'. Similarly, practitioners and teachers may reflect on how they have been shaped by practice and education. Rather than make a singular, authoritative pronouncement on what the mental health nurse is, this book provides a space for 13 authors, drawing on their experience and whatever other sources seem appropriate to them, to address two questions: 'What is your version of the mental health nurse?' and 'How is that nurse trained, educated, found (whatever is appropriate to the version)?'. Contributors to this book were asked to address these two questions, adopting the form and style they thought most appropriate to do so.

Unlike other texts for intending and practising mental health nurses (MHNs), this one presents the voices of these 12 nurses in their variety, without a framing rationale beyond the claim that no authoritative or original legitimating version is available or possible. The basic premise of the book – that it is neither possible nor desirable to produce a single definitive 'version' of the mental health nurse – can be supported in various ways, three of which are now reviewed.

Firstly, the remit of the nurse is now a hotly contested topic. Is the legitimate function and sphere of interest of the MHN now restricted to work with people with long-standing serious mental illness (Gournay, 1995; Barker and Jackson, 1996), or is the wide range of human responses to mental distress the proper focus (Barker *et al.*, 1995)? Should a mental health nurse be instructed in the latest advances in neuropsychiatry and cognitive psychology in order to be able to understand symptomatology and implications for intervention? Or should the MHN become a new kind of 'attendant', practising Buddhism-informed ways of living with and accompanying those seduced by madness (Podvoll, 1990)? Anyone considering becoming a mental health nurse is entering a contested field. She or he will be pushed and pulled in different directions, by texts and teachers, by situated experience, and by self-reflection. Another way to put this is to say that mental health nursing is now plurivocal (many-voiced), not univocal (one-voiced). Many different voices call out to the MHN: do this, learn this, be this way!

Secondly, it is not desirable to give a single authoritative depiction because, insofar as MHNs are concerned with the experience of people in the settings of everyday life, and everyday life is always subject to dispute, mental health nurses must adapt to the circumstances and personalities of the wide world. They could not do so if constrained to use one frame of reference, one repertoire of skills, one delimiting version of reality.

A third way to warrant the book's project is to consider implications of the term 'version' used in describing the aim of the book. The metaphor underlying use of the term is 'mental health nursing as a text'. Mental health nursing is obviously a topic for writers – there are texts about psychiatric nursing. But further implications come from thinking by social scientists, over the past 20 years, about the idea of 'text' as a metaphor for social action. Any kind of social action, including mental health nursing practice, can be regarded as *like* a text. Like a text, action is open to multiple interpretations or readings; action is read in the context of other action, again like texts in relation to a larger canon of literature; and so on. In a related way, insights from the fields of literary theory and criticism become relevant to understanding social action. The idea that there is a fixed text, the true meaning of which readers must try to grasp, gives way to an argument that the reader in some sense creates the text, bringing to inter-pretation of the words on the page background understandings which may be personal or idiosyncratic. Readings may be constrained by unshared, perhaps unsharable background understandings or ideologies.

All of this may seem a fanciful digression from the topic 'the mental health nurse'. It is, however, a central assumption of this book as a whole that there is no single thing to be called 'the mental health nurse' (or 'the psychiatric nurse' – the argument over this distinction is discussed by some of the contributors to this book). Rather, there are different 'versions' of the nurse. Each person coming to mental health nursing can be seen to be like the reader/author of a text, working to grasp and shape the meaning of 'the mental health nurse'. This reader/author is simultaneously the text that is read: the 'I' working to understand the implications of being the nurse. We reflexively construct mental health nursing by participating in it, drawing on our understandings of the field and ourselves in this field.

Writing and reading the book

I chose as contributors people I knew who had already made contributions to literature in the field or who were able to do so, and I judged this through knowledge of their published or unpublished work. This means of selec-tion could make for a very limited book. One could argue that the con-tributors are not representative of the field (in any statistical sense, this is certainly true). Similarly, one could argue that anyone could contribute to a book with the remit outlined. These points are valid, but do not undermine the justification for the book. St. Augustine's saying, 'God is a circle whose centre is everywhere and circumference nowhere', could be translated: mental health nursing's centre is everywhere, its circumference nowhere.

I wanted the book to have some chapters by nurses with long experience of practice and some by nurses new to it; some in practice and others in academic settings and management; nurses with different views on and interests in currently hot and contested topics; those with experience of hospital services and user networks; British, North American and Australasian nurses. All of the authors shared a belief in a plurivocal volume, addressed to intending and practising nurses, representing different versions of the nurse and how she/he is made, and incorporating different views on practice and education. One of the authors is not a nurse and another debates whether he is a mental health nurse (not having that qualification). But all speak to the nurse, on the basis of their experience of and understandings of nursing practice and education.

Readers may seek here a voice that speaks to them, a voice recognisable or attractive in accent, tone or message. They may compare and contrast different versions to see whether all could be accommodated in some incorporating version. They may attend to how these writers construct their versions and their selves in these accounts, and learn something about how as student, practitioner, teacher or researcher they might do something like or different from this. Readers may question the version and imagine what an argument against its claims might be.

My editorial role has been to encourage the contributors to trust their judgement in pursuing these aims. Some of the authors said that they had considerable and, to them, surprising difficulty in writing about themselves and their views. Why this might have been difficult will be discussed in the 'Conclusion'. As editor, I was struck by the commitment they showed to writing their versions. The following summaries are intended to give the intending reader a glimpse of each chapter.

Annie Altschul   Annie Altschul, telling how she came into psychiatric nursing over 50 years ago, argues that psychiatric nurses 'recruit themselves', and that 'people who take to psychiatric nursing are different from those who want to be general nurses'. She then addresses a number of key questions in current psychiatric and mental health nursing. The first is: 'Who are the psychiatric nurses?' She thinks that they have an 'affinity for the underdog'; are 'mature adult people'; 'are fascinated by other people's behaviour, their thoughts and peculiarities'; they 'have considerable inner resources' and 'can be relaxed in silence and inactivity'. Then: 'Who are the patients who need psychiatric nurses?' 'The most severely disturbed people, their families and carers need psychiatric nurses, as do those suffering a variety of other disorders. 'The people who need psychiatric nurses are those who need help, but whom other nurses and many other professionals do not want, or find irritating or frustrating.' To the question 'What do psychiatric nurses do?' she gives Schmalz's reply: 'Drink coffee, smoke and chat', noting that what matters is 'the thinking, feeling and decision making' which goes with these activities. In sum: 'They try to get to know the patient', use self therapeutically, make themselves available, help the patient cope and share everyday life with them. She thinks that psychiatric nurses need to know various matters related to psychiatry and to the care xii The Mental Health Nurse

of people generally, and that 'prolonged contact with different kinds of patients' is essential. Annie thinks that 'because different people recruit themselves', psychiatric nurses should not train or learn alongside general nurses, but may benefit from some learning with other professionals involved with people suffering from psychiatric illness.

Phil Barker and **Irene Whitehill**   Phil Barker and Irene Whitehill present *'our* views ... based on *our* experience of giving and receiving psychiatric nursing'. They begin by exploring the problem of defining 'need' in the context of current UK policy and practice, and the problem of defining nursing. 'Need', they say, implies a requirement for action and a 'lack' which 'constrains the person'. Referring to the etymology of the term, they argue that 'nursing' still connotes 'the process of nourishment' – '[nursing] in contemporary health care' is 'a means of promoting growth and development'. From these considerations of meaning, Phil and Irene turn to the tasks of 'defining the proper focus of nursing', 'developing a discourse on what people need nurses for', and 'discussing how psychiatric nursing might develop while remaining within the nurturing tradition'. They articulate a view of caring as craft – distinct from art or science; '[the] craft of caring ... [implying] that a contractual relationship has been developed between the person-in-care (patient) and the person-who-cares (nurse)'. To explore reflexively the idea that the 'proper focus of nursing ... is on the human development of the service user', they propose to investigate the experience (conveyed in accounts given by *'people-in-care'*) of 'practices which ... promote (or hinder) their growth and development in relation to the experience of illness'. A current project intended 'to clarify the proper focus of nursing' is described. Assumptions held by a group of researchers in Tyneside, about what constitutes psychiatric nursing, are 'illustrated' by Irene's accounts of her 'experiences of nursing' during admissions to hospital and 'care with' a CPN (the ambiguity of 'experiences of nursing' fitting the authors' emphasis on reflexivity and patient–nurse co-operation in the definition of nursing).

Ruth Gallop   Early experience – assignment to a 'difficult patient' – 'hooked' Ruth Gallop into a set of concerns which have driven her career. The concerns centre on understanding aspects of the therapeutic relationship and interpersonal processes, especially empathy; 'working with clients perceived as "difficult"'; and 'working with women'. Ruth's account of 'a personal and professional journey of understanding' explores the interplay between these themes, drawing on a wide range of literature and accounts of her own experience and research. 'Trying to understand the nature of the nurse–patient relationship with patients who are perceived as difficult' entails addressing issues of gender and caring. The power of the relationship is based on empathy; and the relationship is shaped by the mental health nurse's professional role and by the nurse's gender. Ruth considers that '(n)ursing may be a female profession rather than a profession with significant numbers of women'. She argues that the power of mental health nurses and nursing is closely linked to voice. Not only are women patients and difficult patients 'silenced', so too are mental health nurses, the vast majority of whom in Canada are women. The 'voice' of women concerned with 'relational and affective issues' is not heard or is silenced in the presence of the voice of psychiatry. Drawing on Peplau's work, Ruth sees the possibility of 'each new contact' as 'an opportunity for the client to experience connection and engagement...'. As members of a 'disempowered profession', mental health nurses are encouraged to pursue 'personal empowerment' and 'to create a collective voice' to create a 'supportive empowering climate'.

David Glenister   David Glenister challenges 'the assertion that care is the centre of nursing practice', arguing that coercion and control are central in mental health nursing practice. Drawing on various evidence, David addresses a set of topics often not considered in mental health and psychiatric nursing texts: coercion, control, violence, and the use and misuse of power more generally. Coercion is defined as 'the use of legitimated physical force to achieve submission', and control as 'the use of verbal persuasion'. Users' experiences of nurses' coercive and controlling actions are highlighted, as are reports from official inquiries which suggest that 'brutality [and] browbeating' are not relics of mental health nursing's past, but still occur. David discusses associations between race and gender in use of coercion. He argues that 'coercion appears to be more readily applied to black people than to white people', citing 'blindness' to cultural variation, and black people's experience of detention and restraint under the terms of the Mental Health Act. He cites evidence of women's liability to assaults by male nurses. David explores issues of control in the context of changes in mental health service ideology and delivery, and in terms of the impact of invalidation of users' experiences and lived realities. Drawing on psychoanalytical and psychodynamic interpretations, David discusses the role of coercion and control as defence mechanisms protecting nurses from unconscious impulses and anxiety; the organisation of coercion and control; and links between wider economic structures of capitalism and the structure of mental health services. On the basis of this analysis, David recommends that the microsocial, mesosocial, and macrosocial dimensions of 'power' be explored in mental health nurse education, using appropriate kinds of data.

Tessa Parkes   Tessa Parkes has, by her own account, moved 'into, through and beyond psychiatric nursing'. She describes what she sees as tensions in the field, and her struggles as a student and staff nurse to make sense of and to cope with these tensions. Among the issues she explores are the theory–practice gap, and the limited usefulness of theory from other disciplines in helping the mental health nurse understand people's experience of mental distress. Tessa analyses problems of knowledge in mental health nursing, particularly the difference between narrative, interpersonal knowledge ('what it is to be a person struggling in the world') and abstract, decontextualised theoretical knowledge. Listening to patients' stories, 'holding a hand out to [them]', working with them in 'their own unique struggles': these were some of the ways she made sense of and responded to the situations of mental health nursing. Tessa likewise addresses issues of power; the power entailed in labelling and treating others within a diagnostic framework, and in providing an authoritative version of another's experience. Tessa found that 'the most powerful tool I had ... was myself', but also that she was unable to form the kinds of relationship, based on partnership and empowerment, which she wanted to form with patients. Outlining the values and qualities of the voluntary agency she subsequently worked for, Tessa sketches the challenges facing mental health nurses, shaped by work in psychiatric institutions and now in the community (likened to knights roaming the countryside by crumbling castles), as they try to find a place in the current environment of care for mentally ill people.

Linda Pollock   Linda Pollock sketches her career in nursing, from pre-training experience, through work in a poisons unit and community psychiatric nursing and research, to her current position as a Director of Nursing and General Manager of Community Services. She draws lessons from her experiences and educational opportunities, highlighting a number of themes: 'the patient comes first'; the need 'to put the theory of patient care into practice' and to put the patient's emotional and social needs at the centre of nursing interactions; the need for support to articulate experiences and make sense of what one is doing. She conveys her attraction to working with, and the challenge of developing relationships with, emotionally distressed and 'demanding' patients. She outlines the value of the perspective she gained through further training, which focused on understanding patients' needs through developing relationships. Linda describes her own experience of being supported in learning and practice, and her commitment to career-long development of her own and other nurses' ability 'to change situations for the better'. As a manager, she portrays her role in creating opportunities and cultivating a learning climate for staff, and creating a therapeutic *milieu* for patients. Characterising herself as driven by desire for knowledge, she emphasises her support for research to provide proof of effectiveness, the value of 'alternative experiences' in career and personal development, and her determination to ensure that the reason for the National Health Service – caring for patients – does not get lost.

Susan Ritter   Susan Ritter assumes that 'the purpose of psychiatric nursing is mediation, and the management of ambiguity'. The psychiatric nurse 'infers and maintains the boundaries of the internal world of a patient through interpretation of what he or she hears [and] sees', and mediates between this internal world and the outside world. Sue argues that 'in the 1970s and 1980s the education and training of psychiatric nurses combined three incompatible ways of accounting for practice'. The 1982 syllabus for registered mental nurse training promoted questioning of the legitimacy and (im)morality of psychiatric practice, but 'deprive[d] nurses of theoretical principles for organization of their work, for research, and for forming explicit rules for practice in clinical settings'. Arguing that this emphasis risks subverting psychiatric nurses' own claims to legitimacy, Sue asserts the value of testing specific nursing interventions, and questions nurses' 'moral sleight-of-hand' in substituting moral justification for demonstration of clinical effectiveness. Analysing 10 years of psychiatric nursing literature, she notes the limitations of the research base for practice, nurse behaviour therapy excepted.

Dehumanisation of care may stem in part from 'lack of consensus among psychiatric nurses about the formulation of nursing care', legitimating inappropriate warrants for practice: 'Trust me, I'm a nurse'. Sue addresses some implications of the problematic state of psychiatric nursing knowledge, and of participation in health care decision-making. If nurses' 'observation of science remains from the viewpoint of the outsider' they risk compromising their capacity to 'mediate between patients and psychiatry'. Sue draws on her current and past practice, research, and personal experience, and on analyses of nurses' language in 'enforcing/enabling', to develop these arguments. She sketches the 'risks' of trying 'to help a person to reconstitute his or her inner world while retaining his or her individual autonomy'. In managing ambiguity, and helping to restore the patient's 'social being', psychiatric nurses need to be able to 'justify why they rather than anyone else should mediate between the internal worlds of estranged individuals and the outside worlds of which they are necessarily a part'.

Desmond Ryan Desmond Ryan writes, in the first instance, about the hospital nurse. He extends an analysis of the mental health nurse working or learning in the hospital, to consider nurse teachers and researchers. The hospital nurse is, according to Desmond, an ambiguous figure. Adopting the metaphor of the nurse as amphibian – dweller in two realms – he explores dualities in the nurse's role. The nurse is accountable to the hierarchy of authority in the ward, but also responsible to the patient as a person. The ambiguities can be interpreted in 'either-or' terms, in which case the nurse turns towards one or the other of these sources of authority; or in 'both-and' terms. Desmond argues that the best nurses manage the tension of the 'both-and' perspective. The nurse teacher is likewise accountable for the content of lessons, for the purposes of examination and registration; and responsible for a student's development as a person through practice and education. He argues that the best teachers maintain the tension of the 'line' connecting these two roles. The final subject is the researcher. Desmond turns an analytical gaze on himself as interpreter of and writer about nursing. Nurse researchers are accountable in the current health care context, organised by values of science, objectivity, and the 'research and development' project. But the 'amphibian' researcher is also part of the world about which he or she thinks and writes, the subjectively experienced world of persons. Again, Desmond argues that the researcher (and by implication the student learning through research) should maintain the (tension in the) 'line' bridging these two domains.

Duncan Tennant In a chapter describing group work with inpatients in an acute psychiatric setting, Duncan metaphorically visits and re-visits the room in which the group met. The tensions, contradictions and challenges of working in this setting over a 10-year period as a clinical nurse specialist are conveyed from his point of view. Through metaphors of military campaigns and sporting contests, Duncan portrays the issues of power involved in this work. He argues that it entails, for psychiatrists, a 'paradigm shift' in understanding; for patients, challenges of learning through commitment and experience; and, for mental health nurses, living with and resolving the tension between custodial and therapeutic functions. In group work based on interpersonal approaches the nurses and patients have to achieve the conditions necessary to achieve the group's tasks. By extension, achieving the conditions necessary for setting up and running groups is likewise both an interpersonal process and an intrapersonal process. Duncan describes how he looked through a one-way screen to observe the group, and the sudden turn of awareness when he realised the group was 'observing' his observation. Languages of gaze and talk are, he suggests, media through which psychiatrists, nurses and patients negotiate understandings of what they are doing in admission wards. Duncan outlines the knowledge of interpersonal and group dynamics a nurse working in such a setting requires, and indicates the problems, for teachers and students, posed by the current concern to demonstrate outcomes of nursing interventions.

Stephen Tilley Stephen Tilley uses the metaphor of 'the mental health nurse as rhetorician' to explore ambiguities in his own practice, and to interpret current issues in practice and education. Rhetoric is defined as 'the field of knowledge about how to accomplish understanding and avoid misunderstanding', and the art of persuasive speech. Thus skill in rhetoric is useful in resolving competing interpretations to arrive at shared understandings. Stephen outlines the classical view of the rhetorical act as having three aspects: 'proofs', the manner of the speaker, and the emotional response of the audience. He suggests that, while mental health nursing literature has focused mainly on issues to do with 'proofs' or knowledge, the character of the nurse and the desired effects to be produced are vitally important. Stephen argues that mental health nurses' work is unavoidably rooted in common sense. Mental health nurses are concerned with the problems of everyday life faced by their patients or clients; their ability and right to claim specialist expertise is therefore likely to be contested. The rhetorician relates disputes to common topics in a contested common sense. Thus rhetoric is a necessary and valuable tool for mental health nurses who seek to act 'prudently', and to help patients and clients act 'prudently'; to do what is 'called for' in situations where their actions may be called into question. Stephen sees a rhetorical perspective as useful both for understanding the discipline as it is represented in mental health nursing literature, and for preparing the nurse to practise. He emphasises the mental health nurse's obligation to redress unequal power relations in face-to-face interaction with clients or patients.

Christine Walsh Through the theme of 'difference', Christine Walsh explores issues central to the work of New Zealand mental health nurses.

To work with others is to face always the issue of being like and being different from the other. Chris draws on findings from two studies – one illuminating issues of cultural difference, the other describing differences in gender and sexual orientation – to describe implications for the nurse, the client or patient, and the mental health service. She claims that psychiatric nurses are 'trained to expect difference in people; to see it and respond to it appropriately', and that the challenge is to recognise one's own difference as well as that of the other. Differences highlight the ways in which individuals identify with and position themselves in relation to groups. Chris suggests that the emphasis on cost-effective care may jeopardise nurses' ability to work collaboratively with clients in a culturally safe way. Examples based on research and practice with Māori people indicate some of the dimensions of 'culturally safe' and appropriate practice. Chris argues that the experience of New Zealand nurses and patients is relevant to that of mental health service users and providers more generally, insofar as difference is a common theme with particular variations in local settings. She addresses the problems (and possibilities) of writing about a culture other than one's own, and of understanding and responding to people different from oneself. Chris reflexively illustrates how, as a 'Pākehā (white) lesbian woman', she has addressed issues in her practice as a mental health nurse.

Roger Watson Roger Watson poses a fascinating problem: not a mental health nurse, he has spent most of his working life caring for people with mental health problems – elderly people with dementia. This problem of identity has a counterpart in the problem of focus of care for these people. The nurse must compensate for the demented person's deficits in personal, health and social care; indeed, must act for the elderly demented person whose capacities for awareness, thought and communication are profoundly affected. 'The precise nature of the condition is not fully understood', and therefore a rational basis for provision of care is elusive. Roger sketches issues related to where care is provided, and the problem of distinguishing health care need and social care need. Focusing on Alzheimer's disease, Roger describes the main features of the condition which are suitable for a nursing response. Behavioural problems, in particular, fall within the 'domain' of the mental health nurse; but even here, it cannot be argued conclusively that psychogeriatric provision is more appropriate than continuing care. Against the backdrop of these challenges for mental health nurses working with this group of people – questions of definition, remit and effectiveness – Roger describes additional challenges based on 'alternative models of dementia care' and 'new directions in dementia theory'. The new 'optimistic paradigm' in dementia care (focused on the individuality and personhood of dementia sufferers) challenges the 'burden paradigm' (focused on the burden dementia imposes on caregivers). Roger argues that nurses will have to choose between these two incompatible paradigms, and warns against discarding what is of value in current nursing provision.

References

Barker, P. and Jackson, S. (1996) Seriously misguided. *Nursing Times* **92** (34), 56–7.

Barker, P.J., Reynolds, W., and Ward, T. (1995) The proper focus of nursing: a critique of the 'caring ideology'. *International Journal of Nursing Studies* **32** (4), 386–397.

Gournay, K. (1995) Mental health nurses working purposefully with people with serious and enduring mental illness – an international perspective. *International Journal of Nursing Studies* **32** (4), 341–352.

Podvoll, E. (1990) *The Seduction of Madness: A Compassionate Approach to Recovery at Home*. Century, London.

1 A Personal View of Psychiatric Nursing

Annie Altschul

I started general nurse training during the Second World War, in an old 'County' hospital, part of which was still a workhouse. It became clear to me almost at once, that nursing was not for me, but there was conscription for women who were not in essential jobs, so nursing it had to be. I treated it as war work which would come to an end when the war was over. I hated some types of wards more than others. My only experience of surgical nursing was in my very first ward, where I spent my time in the sluice. The operating theatre proved to be impossible and I was employed there, by general agreement, washing up outside. Medical wards were tolerable. Fortunately, the powers-that-be did not bother much about students learning anything new. Once they discovered what you were good at they left you where you were. For me that meant work in the geriatric work-house, on day-night-day-night shifts.

The place had a four-bedded psychiatric 'observation ward'. It was staffed by RMNs (registered mental nurses), but whenever one of them was sick or on leave or whenever they needed help or relief, I was sent there because it was evident to all that I was in my element there. Other places which suited me were a 'casual' ward where tramps spent the night, were examined, bathed, fed and sometimes treated, and a ward called 'Annexe' which was largely used for gypsies, of whom there were quite a lot in the area. Gypsies were considered not to be suitable patients for regular wards. They were regarded so much as inferiors that they were even allowed visitors at all times of the day. It now shocks me to realise that this did not shock me at the time. Clearly my affinity for the underdog was recognised, and my lack of suitability for work in acute wards marked me out for allocation to the wards where underdogs were nursed.

By the time I finished training it was obligatory to work in an area of nursing where there were shortages. Fortunately, psychiatry was one such field of work and I was accepted at Mill Hill EMS Psychiatric Hospital. There I felt at home from the first moment.

I have been convinced, for a long time, that people who take to psychiatric nursing are different from those who want to be general nurses. In this chapter I want to examine what kind of people they might be. I argue that, because different people recruit themselves, psychiatric nurse training and general training should be separate. Generic nurse training does not make sense. Generic training has played havoc with social work; it could do so in nursing.

It is not the curriculum I object to – I have no objection to people learning useless information – but I do object to the attitude of those who do not understand the psychiatric field and who proclaim the unity of the nursing profession. These people believe it to be desirable that every nurse should have what they call 'psychiatric experience', to the detriment of the people who suffer from mental disorder and at the cost of those who want to have in-depth psychiatric training. A short period of experience in a psychiatric ward where severely disturbed patients require specialist care will not, in my view, help any nurse to understand better that some physically ill patients and their friends and relatives can be worried and anxious. This, they should be taught as part of their general experience. Of course, psychiatric nurses should know some facts about physical health, as should all workers, wherever they may function. Food hygiene, prevention of infection, how to protect one's own health (particularly how to prevent back injury if possible), what to do in emergencies and how to recognise when people are physically unwell, are examples. This is certainly important in long-stay geriatric work and in all settings where patients help in the management of the environment of daily living. Some knowledge of nutrition is also useful; however, these topics do not receive much attention in general nurse training and in any case should be part of secondary school education. The overlap of some elements does not justify a generic approach to nursing.

I do not believe that a 'unified nursing profession' is desirable or attainable. Psychiatric nurses have a great deal in common with members of other professions, for example social workers, occupational therapists, youth workers, counsellors, the police and even prison workers; much more than they have in common with nurses in intensive care or in operating theatres.

I should like to examine, in some detail, what kind of person makes a psychiatric nurse, whether one can become such a person if one is not already there on recruitment, and what the implications are for education. I should also like to look at the kind of problems people who need the help of psychiatric nurses have, and what psychiatric nurses do to help them and their carers.

I should like to discuss the topic under five headings:

- Who are the psychiatric nurses?
- Who are the patients who need psychiatric nurses?
- What do psychiatric nurses do?
- What do they have to know?
- How do they learn psychiatric nursing?

These issues are obviously interrelated and will be brought together at the end of this chapter. It helps me and perhaps it will help the reader to think of them separately in the first instance.

Who are the psychiatric nurses?

The first point I should like to stress is that psychiatric nurses are mature adult people. It is not a childhood or adolescent fantasy to aim to become a psychiatric nurse. In fact, I would be suspicious about the motivation of anyone who claimed always to have wanted to become a psychiatric nurse. True, I have met some excellent psychiatric nurses who had made their career choice early in life. Usually they were sons or daughters of psychiatric nurses who had grown up in the environment of psychiatric institutions and been introduced to the work by their parents. Even for these few, however, I think it might have been better if they had gained other work experience first. For most of those I have met, psychiatric nursing was a second career. For some, for myself for example, it was a second choice after qualifying as a general nurse. Many, however, came into psychiatric nursing from the armed services, the police, from social work, community work, from residential care, probation, prison work, from youth work, from having been counsellors, or from careers in sport. People used to joke about those who came from sports careers. They said disparagingly: 'If you have played cricket or football you are in'. I do not believe that the criteria for recruitment were ever as simple as that. I believe, however, that success in a previous career, such as sport, can be a definite advantage. All the good psychiatric nurses I have known had wide interests and deep and extensive knowledge of some field other than nursing. Sport is just one such field, other possibilities are music, arts, poetry and literature. Many are interested in politics, trade unionism and race relations. What many have in common is a commitment to the underprivileged, the poor, the homeless. Many are interested in philosophy, especially ethics, and in anthropology. Their interest in psychology and sociology sometimes antedates entry into the profession, but often arises from their personal contact with patients. I have met psychiatric nurses who have an aptitude for and knowledge of mathematics or of physical and biological sciences, but not any for whom these subjects were the dominant interest.

One important point to make about psychiatric nurses is that there are many men as well as women in the profession. For a long time it was not socially acceptable for men to become general nurses, and it was always very unlikely that school boys would have that ambition, the way school girls often did. But it has always been acceptable that grown men should find themselves attracted to work with people suffering from mental disorder.

Because psychiatric nursing is a field of work where people of both genders mix, it has escaped some of the characteristics of the culture of general nursing, seen as typical of female society. A stereotype commonly associated with women's occupations is that of rigidly hierarchical stratification accompanied by cattiness and subservient behaviour. Perhaps there is some justification for this belief.

For me, it was a liberating experience to have colleagues, both men and women, who led normal lives outside their jobs. Many were married, many had children or elderly dependent relatives. They were people who had no need to protect their rank and status. It was also liberating to escape from the sexual games played out by junior doctors and the nursing staff in the general hospital and to be spared the games in which the predominantly male senior medical staff cast themselves as father figures for 'their' subordinate female nurses.

I am aware that general nursing has changed since the days of my experience. There is more opportunity now for initiative, less adherence to routine. There are more married older women, especially in part-time jobs. Even so, I believe the difference in the kind of people attracted to psychiatric nursing remains.

There are now economic and financial obstacles to the recruitment of mature men into psychiatric nursing. The men who in my opinion would be ideal recruits for psychiatric nursing earn too much money and have too many commitments to consider accepting the salaries which nursing is prepared to offer. Even those made redundant from well-paid jobs could probably not make a living on a psychiatric nurse's starting salary. The other obstacle is the tendency, in nursing, to adhere rigidly to fixed academic entrance qualifications, which older men had neither the desire nor the opportunity to acquire in their youth. That passes in school examinations have no bearing on the ability to learn and that they have no relevance to adult adaptation to work has been amply demonstrated. But at a time when nursing has no difficulty in recruiting well-qualified school leavers there is often a reluctance to modify entrance criteria for mature applicants. It is to be hoped that the move of nursing education into the realm of higher education will encourage nursing to follow the example of universities by exempting mature students from the normal entry requirements.

I have described the interests and the background of the people I think suited to psychiatric nursing. What about their personality characteristics? My experience tells me that psychiatric nurses are people who are fascinated by other people's behaviour, their thoughts, their peculiarities. They are people who are non-judgemental and not easily shocked. They have a fair amount of self-confidence and do not need the gratitude of patients or the admiration of fellow workers. Above all, they are people who have considerable inner resources. Though many are extrovert and enjoy company and social life, others are more content in one-to-one communication. All can be relaxed in silence and inactivity.

Who are the patients who need psychiatric nurses?

This question is not easy to answer. As a nurse I would say that without doubt the most seriously disturbed people, those suffering from schizophrenia, from severe clinical depression or from acute mania, in other words from acute psychotic disorders, need psychiatric nurses. But these terms are categories of medical diagnostic classification, and long before doctors have had a chance to diagnose, sufferers have needed help and relatives and friends have searched for advice and assistance, often baffled by the changed behaviour of their nearest and dearest, often feeling guilty, wondering if they have contributed to the problems, always feeling helpless and misunderstood.

Perhaps if access to psychiatric nurses were available without medical referral, patients and relatives might be helped sooner and more effectively. The patients themselves, however, are sometimes the last people to recognise that they need help. Those suffering from depression often share the opinion others express, that they should try to 'pull themselves together'. Not being able to do so makes them frustrated and increases their feeling of guilt. Those suffering from mania do not understand other people's concern – they feel well, confident and successful. Other people irritate them, especially by implying that they need medical attention for their mental state. Those suffering from schizophrenia are often frightened by their disordered experiences, but insight may well be absent. Neither they nor their close friends gain any comfort from the stigma which is still attached to the diagnostic label of schizophrenia.

Many people, in the early stages of psychotic disorder, seek help for concomitant organic symptoms. General practitioners, physicians and general nurses may well be unsympathetic when they fail to find evidence of organic disorder.

Long-term and chronic disorders

While there is probably some agreement that psychiatric nurses are needed during acute phases of psychotic disorder, the situation is far from clear in long-term and chronic illness. It was fashionable, in the 1960s, to blame nurses for the fact that chronic conditions existed at all. Goffman (1970) wrote as if admission to a psychiatric hospital had caused the patients' problems and as if the staff had been motivated to humiliate and stigmatise their patients. Barton (1976) called the chronic disorder which follows in the wake of acute episodes of psychosis 'institutional neurosis', a term which was less accusatory than Goffman's description and which drew attention to the fact that prolongation of some forms of care deprives patients of initiative. Hospital routine changed for the better as a result of these criticisms, but chronic disorder did not disappear. When the doctors can no longer think of any treatment which might benefit a sufferer from chronic mental disorder, the patient is discharged into 'community care'. Who but psychiatric nurses could help the patient in the community? Relatives and friends do their best, but without professional help they may find the burden too much. Social workers make assessments, but long-term care is often beyond their resources. Those without a supportive network of family or friends certainly need psychiatric nurses for help.

Other forms of mental disorder

How about patients who suffer from other forms of mental disorder? There is a case to be made that people who suffer from phobic disorders, from anxiety states and other severe neurotic disorders can be cared for by psychiatric nurses. During a period of inpatient care the presence of a well-qualified psychiatric nurse may provide a sense of security and enable the patient to regain control. Often psychologists with skills in behavioural therapy are the most effective people to treat such sufferers. Many psychiatric nurses have acquired the necessary skills too. They may be the most appropriate people to help such patients in the community.

There is little evidence to suggest that psychiatric nurses are needed by all the many people who feel that they are under stress because of, for example, problems in their family relationships, their sex life, their work or their physical health.

Do patients suffering from dementia need psychiatric nurses? I find it difficult to decide. On the one hand, their disturbed and sometimes agitated behaviour presents difficulties for nurses other than psychiatric nurses. On the other hand some patients suffering from dementia have a multitude of physical problems for which they require specialist intervention outside the particular competence of psychiatric nurses. It would seem to me that the carers, rather than the patients themselves, may need psychiatric nurses to help them deal with the many problems they encounter.

Psychiatrists are concerned with many more disorders, but whether people suffering from these need psychiatric nurses is difficult to decide. I would be prepared to say that the people who need psychiatric nurses are those who need help, but whom other nurses and many other professionals do not want, or find irritating or frustrating.

Disturbed children

The incidence of psychological disturbances in children is very high (Nicol *et al*, 1993). Many children who might benefit from therapeutic interventions by psychiatrists, psychologists or teachers and health visitors with special skills, are never brought to the attention of such professionals. Often teachers become aware of the difficulties and find suitably qualified professional colleagues to offer treatment. Often parents are left to cope, perhaps with some professional support. A few children are admitted to residential care, in special schools or specialist hospital units. There is always need, in such units, for a multi-disciplinary team. Psychiatric nurses are, in my view, the people who can provide a safe environment and who can create an atmosphere conducive to optimal therapeutic intervention by each member of the team.

People suffering from alcohol or drug dependency

Here too, multi-disciplinary therapeutic intervention is needed. As with children and young people, psychiatric nurses may have a role to play.

People who demonstrate deviant behaviour, those labelled as psychopaths, and those whose behaviour would be dealt with under the criminal justice system but for their psychiatric disorder

In special forensic psychiatric units, nurses have a key role to play and, because of the personality characteristics I have outlined earlier, good psychiatric nurses are possibly the people patients might be able to trust. The patient may regard psychiatric nurses as less threatening than some of the other staff who, in their view, may represent authority.

People with learning difficulties

Some psychiatric nurses have a special interest in work with those who have learning difficulties and they choose to undertake special training to prepare them for this work. The people who need their help may have severe physical disabilities in addition to learning problems. They may also have any of the psychiatric disorders already described, and may range in age from neonates to older persons. The change in terminology in UK legislation (to 'learning difficulties') reallocates their problems from the field of health care to that of education and social work. In so far as they need educational help, they need teachers, not nurses. It may be, however, that because psychiatric nurses are ready to accept people as they are and do not apply value judgements to the intellectual performance of the people they care for, they turn out to be effective teachers. In the past, however, psychiatric nurses have been accused of having expectations which were too low, and of failing to enable their charges to reach their full potential.

What do psychiatric nurses do?

A book written by a German psychiatric nurse (Schmalz 1994) begins with this question, asked by the author's mother. Schmalz's reply was: 'Drink coffee, smoke and chat'. Later she said she had now stopped smoking.

Schmalz's answer summarises well what anyone carrying out a time-and-motion study would find psychiatric nurses doing. The same answer would also perhaps apply to the questions: What does a friend do? What does a mother do? Perhaps even: What does a general practitioner do? What does a manager do? The answer omits any reference to the thinking, feeling and decision making which accompanies coffee drinking and smoking.

I would summarise what psychiatric nurses do thus: they try to get to know their patient. They do it mostly by observing and listening. But what they can observe and listen to is restricted to what the patient offers. What the patient offers is entirely dependent on the nurses' interest in and respect for the patient and on the patient's trust in the nurses. Getting to know the patient cannot be hurried. Knowledge of people develops incrementally, sometimes in the process of observation and listening alone, but more commonly in the process of doing things together, working, playing, eating, learning, drinking coffee together and smoking.

Psychiatric nurses do, alongside the patients, all the things people normally do in their lives. They look after their physical well-being, socialise, indulge in leisure activities, work, shop, garden, clean their homes, decorate, go for walks, spend money, argue, read, study, eat and form relationships.

To be interested in their patients is not difficult for psychiatric nurses; this is what brought them into psychiatric nursing in the first instance. Every moment of contact one has with patients increases the interest in what they think, feel and experience. Nor is it difficult to respect the patients when one realises the enormity of the problems with which they have had to cope, their wealth of experience and the achievements they have accomplished.

The aim of psychiatric nursing is to make oneself available and to assist the patient in developing new coping strategies. To do this it is necessary to know the patient well. Sometimes the nurse has to provide, temporarily, a safe environment in which to experiment. One has to support the patient if he fails, help him recognise his strength and accept his weaknesses. Sometimes one must encourage him to lower the expectations he has of himself. Sometimes one needs to hold up a mirror so that the patient recognises the part he himself has played in the creation of problems and learns to not always blame fate or others. Some patients feel the need to look back over their past and share this with the nurse, others gain more from exploring their experiences of the here-and-now.

During periods of inpatient treatment, the daily life in the hospital, the presence of other patients, the availability of members of staff with professional expertise, and the accepting atmosphere which prevails offer the patient the opportunity to reappraise his life style and to learn new skills. In the community these opportunities have to be created, jointly, by the patient and the community psychiatric nurse.

In the course of getting to know the patient it is inevitable that emotional bonds develop. How to deal with the problems this creates for the patient and for the nurse's own psychological well-being is part of what the psychiatric nurse has to learn; it is also a function of the maturity of the nurse, and a reason why it is important to recruit mature adults.

What do psychiatric nurses have to know?

It seems important that psychiatric nurses should be familiar with the symptomatology of psychiatric disorder, with psychopathology and with medical views about the treatment of psychiatric disorder. Some knowledge about mental health legislation is also necessary. Without such knowledge psychiatric nurses would fail to understand psychiatrists and other workers, would be unable to report to them and to contribute constructively to multi-disciplinary therapeutic teamwork. It is particularly important that they should understand the medical model of mental illness if pharmacological treatment is being used, as they are responsible for administering drugs, monitoring their effect, reporting to the medical staff, and influencing prescribing.

Psychiatric nurses must also know that in many cases it is not at all useful if they base their own approach to patients on the medical model. While psychiatrists are primarily concerned with diagnosis and treatment, nurses are primarily concerned with the patients' experience and understanding of their disorders, and with the patients' ability to cope and to restructure their lives.

Some knowledge of psychology and sociology will be useful. For example, power, helplessness, dependency and stigma are relevant sociological concepts. Poverty and unemployment are important topics, as many patients are unable to work because of their problems, and downward social mobility is for many the outcome of mental disorder.

Conformity and deviance, frustration and aggression seem important psychological topics. An understanding of developmental psychology is of course essential where psychotherapy is practised, whether by the psychiatric nurse or by any other member of the team.

It would be easy to say that psychiatric nurses should have knowledge of anthropology, of politics, of economics and of philosophy as well. But clearly it is impossible to have more than a glimpse of most of these subjects. What nurses must be aware of is that, however much they have learnt, there is a great deal more which they do not know. Each member of the team may have some in-depth knowledge and everyone's expertise needs to be recognised, in terms of what each can contribute to the treatment of the patient and to the education of the team members.

Not only members of the team, but also patients have vast reservoirs of knowledge on which the psychiatric nurse can draw. The expertise patients have acquired in their work experience and their education, the skills they have acquired in membership of various social groups and societies, their hobbies and spare-time interests should not be wasted. Psychiatric nurses have the opportunity to increase their knowledge with every patient they care for. Literature and poetry offer important insights. Every patient's reminiscences, every patient's life story help the nurse to understand psychiatric problems better.

The psychiatric nurse must constantly try to increase self-knowledge. It is every bit as important to recognise one's own strength and weaknesses as it is to recognise those of the patients.

If models for practice seem desirable, the most fruitful ones to choose would come from inter-personal theories and from systems theory. Both these perspectives reveal that it does not matter what background knowledge one brings into an encounter; what matters is how people use each other's contributions and how they incorporate these in their lives.

How can psychiatric nursing be learned?

The academic curriculum should provide a foundation course in the social sciences. Some academic study of mental disorder is required. These courses should span the entire period of psychiatric nurses' professional education and should always be accompanied by work with the patient.

Apart from these two subjects it does not seem to matter very much what is included. In my opinion, no subject is irrelevant. Learning should be shared with students from other disciplines, at the same time as every student becomes socialised into his/her own discipline.

There are people who advocate common core programmes of varying kinds. Currently, in the United Kingdom, all nursing students share a common foundation programme of 18 months before being allowed to take up the branch of nursing of their choice. While this may not do any harm, it seems to waste time, preventing students from immersing themselves in the subjects which are of interest and importance to them. It does not help any of the students to understand each other's work better as they have not yet embarked on their own field of interest. The same reservations apply, I think, to the suggestion which has been made, that doctors and nurses should take some of their courses together. Since the students do not yet know what it is to be a doctor or a nurse, they can hardly be expected to learn to understand both. Shared education becomes much more profitable when each of the students concerned has begun to practise in the chosen field.

I believe very strongly that those who know that they want to become psychiatric nurses should have the opportunity to do so from the beginning, even if, in the end, they choose some of their courses from the general or paediatric nursing syllabus. They should have the opportunity, if they so choose, to take courses with students of social work or any of the other professions, rather than have the offer of nursing courses only. They may prefer to enlarge their knowledge of the arts, literature, computing studies or sciences, rather than study professional subjects of no interest to them.

The practice of psychiatric nursing has to be learnt by having prolonged contact with different kinds of patient. Students have to meet young and old, men and women, professional people, working class people, unemployed people, and white and non-white people. They should meet people of a European background and others. They should work with people suffering from depression, schizophrenia, dementia, phobic disorder, drug dependency and many other problems. It used to be easy to find all of these experiences in mental hospitals. This is no longer so. Even the few patients one may meet in hospital do not stay long enough to provide students with meaningful experience.

The patients who are in psychiatric hospitals are the most severely disturbed and vulnerable people. They need the help of experienced staff, and should not be entrusted to beginning students. Finding areas where students can gain appropriate experience and making optimal use of the limited time students are able to spend in clinical practice alongside an academic course, presents a considerable challenge to those responsible for curriculum planning.

In spite of the view already expressed, that the most vulnerable and seriously disturbed of all patients should not be exposed to inexperienced learners, it is important that students should have some opportunity of being with such patients.

Psychiatric hospital experience should, I think, be late in their course, when they have gained confidence, no longer feel frightened, and have acquired some competence in observational and communication skills. It follows that their early clinical practice must take place elsewhere, for example in nursing homes for the chronically ill, in day centres and in the patients' homes.

If students are not to be taught and supervised by experienced psychiatric nurses in hospital wards, it is of crucial importance that they receive personal supervision, on a continuous basis, from a teacher or mentor who has access to the same clinical areas as the students. In other words, it is essential that the students' academic supervisor shares clinical practice with the students.

At this point it may be useful to itemise learning objectives for clinical practice. These fall broadly into four categories:

- those which relate to the creation of a therapeutic environment;
- those which concern observation, interpretation and reporting of observations;
- communication with a patient, one-to-one, listening, forming a relationship, monitoring the effect of this on the patient and the nurse; and
- communicating with patients in a group setting and dealing with relationships between members of the group.

My experience in the USA showed that emphasis was placed mainly on the third of these four areas. Students learned to form and maintain a relationship with one patient and, in weekly sessions with their mentor, learned how to use this in a therapeutic way. It was impressive to observe how much insight the student gained into their own personality and how soon they become aware of the extent to which the patient's behaviour was a response to the student's own actions. The mentor's supportive, non-judgemental attitude was the key to success. The mentor, in turn, relied on the support of a peer group.

My view is that this aspect of the psychiatric nurse's work is only one part of her/his function, and that for many patients it is not the most important one. Sharing the patient's daily life, wherever that may be, observing and communicating in the course of other activities, piecing together a picture of the patient from fragments of information obtained as a by-product of activities, is in my opinion every bit as important.

Psychiatric nursing cannot be learned without exposure to people suffering from psychiatric disorder, but some components of it can be learned without recourse to health service agencies. Participant observation, for example, does not, in the first instance, have to be learned with patients. It can be practised in groups of students, in the cafeteria, in the social centre, in the course of a seminar. Observation of people's behaviour and interpreting the meaning of it can be rehearsed through role play. Significant episodes of disturbed behaviour can be recorded on audio- or video-tape and discussed with fellow students. People with very disturbed behaviour can be seen in the street, the parks, the supermarket, in cinemas and in restaurants. All experiences in the community can be exploited in education.

The incidence of psychiatric disorder is so high that most students are likely to have experienced it in their own circle of family or friends. They should be encouraged to talk about this with each other and their teachers, without feeling embarrassed and without feeling guilty about managing less well in their own lives than in their dealings with patients. It is important for students to learn that, in their professional roles, they may become parent figures, friends, confidants, that patients may see them as substitute sons or daughters, bosses or teachers. Their professional roles are, however, different from real family or social roles. In real role relationships there are reciprocal rights and obligations. Friends and families make demands on each other. Patients are entitled to make demands on nurses whom they see in the role of a parent, but the nurse can not make demands on the patient.

An understanding of the difference between professional and natural social roles will make it easier for students to deal with their emotional reaction to patients and to deal with what is sometimes referred to as 'getting involved'. The student must be helped to deal with the recurring experience of getting close to patients and then suffering the pain of having to break off the relationship again. If the student does not get support in this, there is a danger of either keeping closeness a secret from the team, and therefore not being able to use it therapeutically, or of avoiding closeness altogether, becoming immune to feelings.

One cannot change from natural to professional roles with one's family or friends. This is why carers have particular problems when they have to deal with unacceptable behaviour of those they love and why they need the support of a psychiatric nurse who can maintain a professional role.

A personal note

This chapter started on a personal note. I should like to finish in the same vein. In spite of the editor's use of the term 'mental health nurse' in the title of the book, I have referred to 'psychiatric nurse' throughout. I was sorely tempted to write 'mental nursing'. I am a RMN, a registered mental nurse. No apology is needed. 'Mental' is not a dirty word; it has a respectable etymology, it refers to the mind. To have a mental disorder is no more shameful than to have a bodily disorder.

It has always seemed regrettable to me that the term 'mental' has gone into disfavour with the public and with mental nurses themselves. Why was it necessary to introduce what appears to be a euphemism? How can nurses adopt, officially, the point of view that mental illness is no different from other illnesses, when they themselves shy away from using the word 'mental' about their patients and about their own profession? However, the word 'psychiatric' has entered into everyday vocabulary so I accepted it for my own qualification. Recently this word seems to have acquired a pejorative connotation. 'Psychiatric' is being banished, 'mental health' is the 'in' phrase.

I absolutely refuse to accept 'mental health nursing' for several reasons. The first one of these is that I know nothing at all about mental health, nothing about how to promote it, nothing about protecting it. I do not think many people know what mental health means. The second reason is that nursing intervention is not normally required until health is threatened or lost. I think I understand how health visitors promote health, but I cannot imagine what mental health nurses might do. Thirdly, as a citizen I resent the idea that nurses should take it upon themselves to intervene in my life when I am healthy; and as a taxpayer, I resent training and employing nurses to minister to the healthy, when so much suffering should be alleviated.

In my introduction I said that the five topics of psychiatric nursing are interrelated. My discussion should perhaps have begun with the second section, the patients who need to be nursed. The term 'patient' is used here advisedly. I object to the use of 'clients' in place of 'patients'. If those who need help are no longer patients, then, by definition, nurses are redundant. Nurses and patients have reciprocal roles. What precisely it is that constitutes the nurse's role in respect of any one patient is what I have attempted to show under topic three. Of course, the patient's expectations of the nurse may not always coincide with the nurse's assessment of the patient's nursing needs. Some patients associate the term nurse with physical care and may fail to appreciate the services the nurse has to offer.

In discussing what nurses do I have tried to show that psychiatric nursing has low visibility. It is especially difficult to make visible what the nurse does to create a safe environment, how a therapeutic atmosphere is provided, how anxiety is calmed, how violence is prevented. The nurse's role in providing 'custodial care' is denigrated by the public and by the professions; the nurse's skills are largely unrecognised until a crisis occurs. Patients and other nurses may think that the fact that psychiatric nurses remain calm in tense situations indicates a lack of concern. I asked whether the personality characteristics of a good psychiatric nurse can be acquired or whether they are prerequisites for the job. I hope to have shown, in the last section of my discussion, that the nurse's personality is developed and enhanced by inter-personal relationships with each patient and in each encounter within the inter-disciplinary team. Supportive supervision is an essential component in the development of professional integrity.

The manner in which psychiatric nurses apply their skills is referred to in the literature as 'the therapeutic use of self'. This concept is best described by Peplau (1988). A full discussion of it is beyond the scope of this chapter. It is an important concept, however, and I would like to refer to it in this last section.

What makes psychiatric nursing so interesting is the constant endeavour to use one's 'self' therapeutically, for the benefit of the patient. Every success, however small, is immensely gratifying. On the other hand, knowing how little influence one really has on other people's lives prevents a feeling of self-importance and self-satisfaction.

Prolonged intensive constructive work in a one-to-one relationship is very stressful, for the patient and the nurse. The time may come, after many relationships with patients, when the nurse no longer feels able or willing to continue. The fifth topic dealt with this issue. Psychiatric nursing is often chosen as a second career. It does not have to be the last one. The knowledge and skills acquired in psychiatric nursing can be usefully applied in other fields of nursing or in other occupational spheres.

Having made a case for the separation of psychiatric nursing from other branches of nursing, I end by recommending post-registration generic advanced professional development and some form of higher education in which previous achievement is accredited and from which new opportunities can open up.

References

Barton, R. (1976) *Institutional Neurosis,* 3rd edn. J. Wright, Bristol.

Goffman, E. (1970) *Asylums.* Penguin, Harmondsworth.

Nicol, R., Strech, D. & Fundudis, T. (1993) *Preschool Children in Troubled Families. Approaches to Interventions and Support.* John Wiley & Sons, Chichester.

Peplau, H.E. (1988) *Interpersonal Relations in Nursing.* Macmillan, London.

Schmalz, U. (1994) *Rette Mich Wer Kann.* Psychiatrie-Verlag, Bonn.

2 The Craft of Care: Towards Collaborative Caring in Psychiatric Nursing

Phil Barker and Irene Whitehill

Caring: first principles

Psychiatric nursing is predicated on the twin assumptions that there are such 'things' as psychiatric needs, and that nursing might in some way meet those needs. Here, we hope to discuss what these needs might be, and how psychiatric nurses might begin to meet them. A useful starting point might be, therefore, a reconsideration of what we mean by 'needs' and 'nursing'.

The concept of need

The popular parlance of health care provision of the 1990s has been dominated by all sorts of consideration of need. To borrow Stephen King's (1991) phrase, the 'needful things', for which we offer services to patients [*sic*], may carry some kind of unknown penalty in their wake. The idea, for example, that we shall endeavour to meet the 'individual and unique' needs of the patient, casts her/him very much as an 'individual', separate from family, friends, culture and society.

Services which do not purport to be 'needs-led' will be 'needs-driven', in either case necessitating 'needs-assessment' or an 'assessment of need'. Whether or not there is any consensus on the nature of such needs remains unclear. In our view a 'need' is something which requires action. Despite the commonly expressed distinction between a 'need' and a 'want', both expressions convey the sense of 'lack' or 'deficiency' which, in practical terms, constrains the person. People might need or want more money, more stability, more friendship, more comfort or whatever.

The professional stance that 'we cannot give everyone what they want' may reflect the practical impossibility of attempting to respond to all healthcare needs or wants. This does not, however, diminish the subjective truth of the person's need. The professional position also implies a moral stance: that some people should not need to express such wants. It also implies that psychiatric professionals might legitimately decide what people in their care 'really' need. It seems self-evident that a major conflict exists between the various 'charters' published by the British government, which claim to assure rights of access to health care, and the distribution (doling) process whereby we are obliged to share out health care resources. (A number of 'charters' have been published by the British government, each of which represents an effort to guarantee certain rights to the citizen. One such charter, The Patient's Charter, identifies what services, and level of provision, people might expect from the health care system.)

It is noteworthy that the archaic expression 'dole' meant 'grief, sorrow or lamentation'. Were it not for the unfortunate association of the term with unemployment benefit, 'dole' would be the most appropriate word to describe the process of needs-meeting. Increasingly, both professional and political commentators argue that we shall never be able to meet all the mental health needs of the population; the non-sequitur being that only the needs of the most seriously distressed or disadvantaged should ever be met. How we define these needs, or the people who have them, remains unclear. Indeed, it has become commonplace to interpret 'serious mental illness' as meaning only 'schizophrenia'. By implication all non-psychotic forms of mental illness are 'minor' (see Gournay, 1995).

It is also noteworthy that the re-focusing of health care on people with 'serious or enduring mental illness' has resulted in the relegation of people with all other forms of 'mental illness' to something near pariah status. Despite psychiatric nurses in the United Kingdom having redefined themselves as 'mental health nurses' they have been encouraged increasingly to re-dedicate themselves to the needs (only) of people with 'serious and enduring mental illness' (Department of Health, 1994).

The situation is complicated further by the realisation that there is a difference between an 'expressed need' and a 'felt need'. People who 'need' mental health services, and perhaps also their carers, may find it extremely difficult to express exactly what their 'needs' are, and might need to be empowered to do so.

Many service users do not know what currently is on offer or what potentially might be available to them. Often the person's decision-making skills may have become depleted, if only temporarily. They may be in awe of professionals whom they believe 'know best'. Their overall expectations of the service may be low and they may be frightened to challenge what they perceive to be 'authority'. Where people have only ever experienced one particular service they have nothing to compare it with.

An everyday example of 'limited experience' might serve to illustrate the dilemma raised here: the use of duvets versus blankets. The nursing team on a long stay ward wanted to offer the people in their care the choice of having a duvet instead of blankets. None of the patients had used one before so could not make an informed choice. The staff offered a trial run of a week, after which people could choose one or the other. Problem solved. Through this simple gesture the people were empowered to express their needs.

Service users recognise that there is a finite amount of money available for planning, developing and delivering services. However, this should not prevent them from expressing their needs, even when these might not be met by the existing services. Service users, and their needs, should not be expected to 'fit' into a static system. Rather, services should be reviewed continuously, in an effort to re-shape or re-orientate the service to meet the users' needs better.

User involvement in care planning, especially in the British system called the Care Programme Approach (CPA), is based on the principle that people using the service should be empowered in such a way that their 'needs' can be better expressed and met. Of course, there will always be some 'unmet need'. This should, however, be documented and used in future planning of services. People should be enabled to take an active role in decision-making. They need to be able to work as equal collaborators.

With the advent of advocacy schemes and user involvement projects, it might be assumed that the only people with any responsibility for promoting the needs of service users are independent advocates, advocacy workers or user involvement workers. Far from being viewed as promoters of personal growth and development, nurses may all too often be seen as representatives of 'the system' which controls those in its care through the wielding of organisational and interpersonal power. Nurses need to reclaim, immediately, their role in the empowerment process. If they do not they will lose the hard-earned skills necessary for the fulfilment of this vital aspect of health care provision. If nurses are to promote the process of identifying and meeting people's needs, they need to recognise that, although they are not advocates *per se*, nursing supports the development and expression of the advocacy process, whereby people's needs and wants are identified.

The concept of nursing

All the indications are that the term 'nursing' denoted a significant function (or important functions) of interpersonal behaviour, long before it acquired the more restricted sense which we associate with (even) the earliest forms of nursing practice, and the emergence of more modern forms of the discipline of nursing (see Barker, 1989). As an enduring human interpersonal activity, nursing involves a focus on the promotion of growth and development (Barker, 1995). The term 'nursing' derives from French *nourice* and the Latin *nutritia*, words meaning the process of nourishment. In English, the term has come to embrace a wider range of meanings, without straying too far from the original.

When people are described as 'nursing a beer' (or any other alcoholic drink) it is implied that they are drinking 'carefully' and slowly, in an effort to prolong an activity deemed, in that culture, to be worth maintaining. Athletes are 'nursing an injury' when they adopt a restrained (or careful) style of movement, to prevent the exacerbation of the injury, or (by taking care) return the injured part to its normal function. More extravagant metaphors are found in forestry where the forester plants a sapling in the shade of an established tree so that the 'infant' tree may gain shelter from the elements, thereby promoting its chances of growing and developing.

The forester talks of 'nursing the sapling'. When, in table billiards, the player uses a particularly 'careful' stroke (characterised by gentle actions) which increases his chances of achieving a high score, the billiard player is 'nursing the balls', exercising care, attention and the minimum of force required to move the balls around the table. This style of play is to be distinguished from the more forceful 'potting' of balls or 'power play' exhibited often by the snooker player .

In everyday parlance, the sense of nursing as a means of promoting or maintaining some treasured 'thing' or 'quality' is conveyed in a number of expressions: 'nursing one's delphiniums' – taking special care to promote growth and development; 'nursing one's strength' – using it sparingly to maintain a reserve; and 'nursing a cold' – trying to cure by taking 'care'. We even recognise nursing as a capacity to keep a thought or feeling alive in our minds, for example 'nursing a grudge' (Watson, 1968).

These metaphorical reference points can help clarify the meaning of nursing in contemporary health care. They suggest the potential of nursing as a means of promoting growth and development, even where damage and disease is readily apparent. Defining nursing (merely) as 'what nurses do', is not without its complications. The catalogue of abuse in mental hospitals in England (especially) during the 1960s and 1970s attests to the inhumanity which may be practised by those called 'nurses', but which has nothing whatsoever to do with the theory and practice of nursing.

As we write, nurses are 'extending their roles' to accomodate drug-prescribing privileges [sic] and are beginning to take over some of junior doctors' diagnostic responsibilities. These developments illustrate the use of people called nurses within health care systems. Whether or not pre-scribing and diagnosing constitute part of nursing is open to question. We intend to adopt a more fundamental approach to defining the proper focus of nursing. Our interest is in developing a discourse on what people need nurses for. This may reveal the unique need for nursing, as distinct from a need for care by doctors, psychologists, social workers, etc. We are inter-ested in discussing how psychiatric nursing might develop while remaining within the nurturing tradition suggested by the root definitions, nourice and nutritia.

Caring – art, science or craft?

Nursing has been described as an interpersonal activity for at least the past 40 years (Peplau, 1952). More recently there have been attempts to reclas-sify this activity within a quasi-scientific paradigm. Many commentators have discussed the art and science of nursing and others have suggested that there might even be a 'science of caring' (Watson, 1989). Here, we discuss what might be described as an alternative paradigm of nursing: nursing as craft, an activity which is not specifically an art or science, but might have some of the elements of each. Given the inherent distinctions between any art and a science, we are unsure how nursing could be both, at least at one and the same time.

Art and science

The process of producing a work of art involves making a creative statement, and is usually conducted in isolation. The resultant creative statement also stands alone. The person who 'appreciates' the artwork does not modify it any way; at least not without risking constructing a pastiche of the original. Artists make a statement and others appreciate that statement: end of story.

The scientist either explains a phenomenom, using scientific theory; or applies this body of knowledge to some problem, constructing a solution. (This latter is often called technology and may be viewed as an 'inferior' form of science). People use the scientist's construction, whether this takes the form of some product, invention or even a marketed idea. Psychotherapy might be an example of psycho-technology: principles which are based on studies of some people, from which core characteristics are abstracted and 'marketed' for consumption by other people. People use or consume the products of science in the same way they consume the products of art; they cannot change or modify them, without risking reinventing or bastardising the product.

The craft process

The craft process appears to be different. Craft is based on an implicit contractual relationship between the craftsperson and the consumer of the craftwork. Craft involves a product which has a function, but no inherent 'meaning': usually it conveys no specific emotion. Any meaning ultimately associated with the craftwork is given by the user. A jeweller makes a ring which may be regarded as aesthetically pleasing. The ring has, however, no meaning of itself. This meaning is given by the wearer of the ring, who transforms it into a symbol of attachment, an heirloom or something of sentimental value, through *use* of the ring. Potters make and decorate, but the users determine specific uses for the pots, attributing meaning in the process. The same process is involved in the wearing of crafted clothing, often seen as a projection of the wearer's personality.

The term 'art' suggests that the product is complete and bounded by the creative experience of the artist: the artist gives the meaning to the work; or somehow draws out (abstracts) the meaning from the artwork, whether visual, literary or musical. The same seems true of scientific 'findings'. Mozart's music or the theory of relativity may hold different kinds of significance for each of us, but we do not bestow meaning on these 'works': *they* enlighten *us*. Craft appears to be different, in the sense that each owner makes the piece special to them: they attach personal significance to the craftwork. A ring may carry similar 'general meanings' but will be given 'specific meanings' by the wearer. A ring worn on a specific finger is interpreted, within certain cultures, as a sign of betrothal. What 'getting engaged or married' means will, however, differ from one person to the next. When the ring is translated into an heirloom – 'this was my grandmother's engagement ring' – additional layers of meaning and significance are attached, thereby changing again the meaning of the ring-craft.

The craft of care

What happens if we extend these metaphors to the 'caring' scenario? Some 'caring' interactions appear to be artistic. When the nurse holds the hand of a person in pain, whether physical or emotional, this gesture, which might be termed a performance, may well be accepted as a complete compassionate 'gift' which the person appreciates for what it is (its essence). Knowing *where* to hold someone (anatomically) might involve the application of some 'science'. Alternatively some nursing interactions appear to be 'scientific', or at least technological, when the nurse uses a knowledge of anatomy and physiology to introduce a drug into a tissue with the minimum of discomfort. How the nurse speaks to the person, perhaps distracting the patient [sic] during the execution of a potentially distressing procedure, might involve the practice of a discrete art. These examples show how the practice of care might oscillate between art and science. Such care is not, however, specific to nursing and may be enacted by other health care disciplines, and even voluntary 'carers' of people with physical or mental distress.

We assume in this discussion that the 'craft of caring' implies that a contractual relationship has been developed between the person-in-care (patient) and the person-who-cares (nurse). We do not aim to demonstrate here the validity of this concept, far less to prove it, but rather assume that whatever 'provides the necessary conditions for the promotion of growth and development' *is* nursing and that which does not is *not* nursing. This view is an echo of Peplau's original assertion that nursing was a 'developmental activity' (Peplau, 1952). If the proper focus of nursing (Barker *et al.*, 1995a) is on the human development of the service user, then further clarification of nursing may emerge from examples provided by 'people-in-care' themselves, who can describe their experiences of practices which appeared to promote (or hinder) their growth and development in relation to the experience of illness.

Caring: finding the proper focus of nursing

The risk of deindividuation

The experience of mental illness has a distinctive quality, invariably linked to the person's identity. The experience often (if not always) appears to involve the whole of the person. People may talk as if they have diabetes, cancer or hypertension, but the experience of depression, schizophrenia or mania is often described as if the disorder has taken over the person. Hence the popular medical convention of talking about people as if they were 'neurotics', 'schizophrenics' or 'personality disorders'. As Wright (1991, p. 481) noted, although diagnostic manuals alert psychiatrists to the risk of diagnosing the person rather than the disorder, the process of 'losing the individual within the group [which Wright calls 'deindividuation'] is so insidious that all too readily it reaches the ultimate point of dehumanisation – the person is then made equivalent to the mental disorder'.

People in mental distress have often been characterised as 'alien': having experiences which are not simply exaggerations of 'normal' experience, but of a wholly different order. Some people *in* mental illness show no overt signs of illness but are thought to 'give themselves away' through their behaviour. The popular fear of the mentally ill – that they are not all that they seem – may have something to do with society's attribution of 'non-human' or 'other' status to all forms of mental ill health, but especially psychosis – 'real madness'. Although this may say more about those who make such distinctions than about whether such distinctions are valid, the abstract, or invisible, nature of mental illness contributes an enigmatic, and threatening, dimension to the social perception of the problem. However, since psychiatric nursing is focused, primarily, on the mental life of the person, and is required, therefore, to accommodate all the *human* considerations noted already, psychiatric nurses have special responsibilities. We might even say that these considerations confer on psychiatric nursing a special status. Psychiatric nursing's focus on problems of identity and experience distinguishes it from those branches of health care which promote the healing of manifest wounds (surgical nursing) or measurable growth in children (health visiting).

Making sense of mental illness

It is important to note, at this point, that we believe that mental illness does exist. However, we think that it is unhelpful to subscribe to the assertion that it is a biological phenomenon, or a manifestation of political dispossession, or some equally reductionist explanation. Whatever it is that ails people when some say that they are mentally ill (or, as we would prefer to say, are in mental illness), is far too complex for such simplistic forms of categorisation. It is more important to *understand* what might be going on when people experience what is described as mental illness, than to classify or categorise either the experiences, or the person concerned. If we are to develop a craft of care in psychiatric nursing then we need to know what the experience of mental ill health *means* to the person who is 'in' that experience.

Porter (1987, p. 232) took the view that the mad [*sic*]:

> 'make sense with that very universe of language, metaphor, idiom and symbols which the sane themselves articulate. The mad talk about fathers and mothers, about God and kings and devils, about shock waves and inspiration just as the sane do, though the nuances are different.'

It would be foolish to assume that the sane have a monopoly on reality and truth (whatever these terms mean). Porter (1987, p. 232) noted that the sane and the mad share similar territories of experience:

'We all have phantoms in the head. Each act of conception, each account, analysis, stab at historical understanding, is an expression of our preconceptions, every bit as much as it may be (we hope) a brick of truth. It also brings out our prejudices. It would be self-deluding to pretend that these do not exist.'

Porter's views may convey something of the sense of Sullivan's (1953) dictum that 'we are all more alike than different'. Indeed, experiences common to all, such as dreaming, are akin to psychosis, undercutting the view that the more severe or serious forms of mental illness, such as psychosis, are somehow beyond normal experience.

Towards a definition of the proper focus of nursing

Theoretical formulations of nursing have been developing steadily over the past 40 years. Most available theories and models do not focus specifically on the unique context of psychiatric nursing care. We would like now to discuss current work in a British setting which aims to clarify the proper focus of nursing (Barker *et al.*, 1995a), through research which reflects on the distinct and mutual experiences of caring as described by nurses and the users of nursing. The following premises derive from current work by the Tyneside Group (Barker *et al.*, 1995b; Barker & Stevenson, 1996).

We propose that psychiatric nursing is based on the following four core premises. Each is illustrated briefly with examples from one co-author's (Irene's) experience of being nursed.

Premise 1
Psychiatric nursing is an interactive, developmental, human activity, more concerned with the future development of the person than with the origins or causes of their present mental distress. Therefore, psychiatric nursing is concerned to establish the conditions necessary for the promotion of the person's unique growth and development. Such growth and development will, of necessity, involve the person's adjustment to, or overcoming of, the life-problems associated with mental illness.

It is essential to deal with the life-problems associated with mental illness so that people can get on with their ordinary lives outside of the health care system. This does not preclude the exploration of possible origins of triggers for mental distress. Such exploration is an aid to moving forward, rather than becoming locked in the past, an all too common experience for some people.

Whilst receiving cognitive therapy from a nurse Irene looked at the possible triggers for her mania:

'The 10 episodes which required hospitalisation occurred at times when I was under stress due to over-work and difficulties with sexual partners. Through cognitive-based counselling I developed a greater awareness of these potential triggers and have tried to alter my life style accordingly. This heightened awareness has enabled me, on a number of occasions, to recognise the early symptoms of mania, and to prevent a full blown episode by taking the requisite medication. Quite often I recall the discussions we had in those sessions.

During the past 15 years I have had many discussions with community psychiatric nurses (CPNs) about my "over-working" and how to manage it. However, my current CPN is the best one I have had. She actually has the courage to "read the riot act" to me about my "over-working". Further, we have discussed ways by which I could maintain a better balance in my life and the difficulty of managing periods of creativity.

Ours is very much an equal relationship. We have built up a good rapport and in different circumstances I feel that we could be good friends. I only see her when I feel in need of support. It gives me confidence to know that I can opt in and out of a service as I choose. I feel in control, being able to negotiate times when she will call. She acts as my sounding board, helping me make decisions and think through problems. Rarely does she offer advice unless I encourage her to do so. Sometimes we just chat about books, holidays, my work and involvement with the church.

She supported me in sorting out my finances last year when I had three hospital admissions and was not able to work for several months. It was difficult to face the bank manager at a time when I was very much lacking in confidence. She gave me that extra bit of courage I needed to don my "power dressing" jacket and to "strut my stuff". We have also discussed a bi-polar management chart to help me spot more quickly the onset of hypomania.

Last year, when in hospital, I tried, without much success, to convince my psychiatrist that I needed a befriender or enabler to help me for a few weeks when I got home. Thanks to my CPN, who is also my care manager, I got a part-time home help for a 6-week period after coming home from hospital.

Second only to the course of cognitive therapy, this is the best example of practical help I have received from the mental health services. It enabled me to catch up with the back-log of paperwork which had accumulated during my stay in hospital, without worrying about the housework. This was a great relief as I am extremely tidy and it affects my whole mood if the flat is in a mess.

On discharge from hospital you lack confidence and take longer to do things. It's difficult to know where to start. Simple things seem very difficult and easily get on top of you. I liken myself to a new-born lamb struggling to find its feet. My relationship with my current CPN is definitely an example of "caring with" rather than "caring for". I can discuss with her issues that I possibly wouldn't with a friend, because we are not "associated"'.

Premise 2

The experience of mental distress associated with psychiatric disorder is represented through public behavioural disturbance, or reports of private events, but is known only to the individual concerned. Psychiatric nursing involves the provision of the necessary conditions under which people may access and review those experiences. Such collaborative re-authoring of the person's life might involve the healing of past distress and the opening of ways to further human development.

In Irene's view it would be a novel idea if nurses listened to the total experience of service users, as seen through their own eyes:

'It would validate the person's experience. It would offer them an opportunity to share their own interpretations, seek explanations, and diffuse any fears or guilt, and feelings of anger or bewilderment. It might also serve to challenge our concept(?s) of reality, sanity and insanity. Thinking of *Gulliver's Travels* we might well ask, "whose reality is it anyway?"

Service users are often punished by the system. They are forced to collude with mental health professionals in the suppression and denial of their experiences. Therefore, these experiences become stigmatised, and by extension, the person is stigmatised.

In seeking counselling or psychotherapy, many service users are merely trying to repair the damage caused by this stigmatisation. This situation will be perpetuated for as long as mental health professionals continue to disregard the personal meanings events have for the people in their care.

Eleven of my thirteen admissions to hospital have been precipitated by manic episodes. During each episode I heard voices, had visions and was aware of presences. Many of the episodes had religious connotations. On three occasions I believed that I was another person – the Virgin Mary, Emily Pankhurst and Wayne Sleep. My desire to be a nun, deaconess or trainee chaplain was apparent in several of the episodes. Two of the episodes were associated with the national miners strike and the threatened redundancy of 30 000 miners. In a recent episode, I experienced a very powerful transference experience.

Whilst in hospital I was never encouraged to discuss these episodes. The phrase, "it's just part of your mania" has been quoted at me on numerous occasions. Since many of the episodes held religious significance to me I have spoken with a number of clergy. All but one, I felt, listened and accepted although they could not always offer a clear explanation. During my first episode, when I believed that I was the Virgin Mary, my local vicar refused to talk to me about it and virtually chased me away from his church.

Thankfully, over the past 15 years I have met a great many service users who have had similar experiences. Although this is reassuring I remain concerned that we are not enabled to talk openly with mental health professionals about our experiences. On the one hand, I feel privileged to have had these experiences, which have been of great significance in my life. On the other, I feel stigmatised, as professionals associate my experiences with "the illness" and not my general life experience. I regard all 13 of my "nervous breakdowns" as periods of spiritual transformation which have resulted in a spiritual crisis. These crises, which all happened at significant times in my life, were enriching experiences and resulted, very much, in personal growth.

Whose reality is it anyway? The visions, presences and voices I experienced during my manic episodes were "real". In between episodes, when I am experiencing good health, I still hear voices and experience presences. They are just as "real".

Some people hold the belief that different realities exist in different planes, at the same time. Similarly, different levels of consciousness may be attained, for example through meditation. The presences and voices which I experience when I am "well" may be God, people who are known to me, or strangers. If they are of people currently known to me I am often tempted to ask the individuals whether or not they are aware of our conversations taking place. Are they telepathic or is this an example of reality on another plane?

Far from being seen as a symptom of mental illness, being able to hear voices is viewed in some cultures, for example Native American Indian and African cultures, as a form of spiritual communication, and regarded as a "gift" from God. Those who hear voices, shamans, are heralded as spiritual leaders. People can be enabled to develop the "gift" through various spiritual practices. Likewise, Christians believe that they can tune into the voice of God through prayer, meditation and fasting. I believe that during prayer and at other times I am in direct conversation with God.'

Premise 3
The nurse and the person-in-care are engaged in a relationship based on mutual influence. It is assumed that the reflexive nature of the caring experience produces changes for the nurse, the person-in-care, and significant others. Nursing involves caring with rather than caring for people, irrespective of the context of care.

'I very much favour the concept of nurses caring "with" rather than caring "for" people. "With" implies a partnership, shared responsibility for the caring process; an equal relationship. "Caring with" enables the service user to take an active part in their own care. "Caring for", on the other hand suggests an unequal relationship. The service user is forced to maintain a passive role in the caring process. The relationship is unequal, since the nurse is holding the power.

At present I am served by a rehabilitation team. My current CPN is the best nurse I have had and exemplifies the notion of "caring with" people. Her style of nursing is extremely empowering. She treats me very much as an equal and is never overly supportive. I value her support in working through problems and making decisions. She has encouraged me to self-manage and take responsibility for my own medication.

During a recent hypomanic attack we worked together to identify how much medication I required. As a result I was able to manage the episode over a period of a week. We worked out a step-wise dosage regime to which I adhered and the episode subsided. I knew that I could contact her at any time during the week and additional support was arranged at the weekend.

Her level of involvement with me varies depending on how much support I need. We have built up a great deal of trust which means that I have no hesitation in contacting her when I need support. She recognises my high level of insight and always enables me to decide when her next visit should be. After 15 years in the system this is extremely refreshing!

Our relationship is very much two-way. I know that I have challenged her perception of a mental health service user, whilst influencing her thinking on the management of manic depression and a number of other mental health issues. Our relationship could be summed up by these lines from a poem entitled *Listen* (Anon., cited in Bauer & Hull, 1986):

When I ask you to listen to me
and you start giving advice
you have not done what I asked

When I ask you to listen to me
and you begin to tell me why I shouldn't feel that way
you are trampling on my feelings

When I ask you to listen to me
and you feel you have to do something to solve my problem
you have failed me, strange as that may seem.

When you do something for me that I can and need to do
for myself, you contribute to my fear and weakness.

So, please listen and just hear me. And, if you want to
talk, wait a minute for your turn; and I'll listen to you.'

Premise 4

*The experience of mental illness is translated into a variety of disturbances of
everyday living. The practice of psychiatric nursing is located uniquely within the
context of everyday life. As a result nursing care is invariably an in vivo activity:
focused on the person's relationship with self and others within the context of their
interpersonal world. Nursing practice is focused on helping people address their
human responses to mental illness, rather than the illness itself which is, by definition, a professional construct.*

'I agree that mental health nurses could fulfil an important role in helping people
address their human responses to "mental illness". Service users are repeatedly
stigmatised by the system and the society within which they are trying to develop
"ordinary" lives. Consequently, they feel punished and devalued, often developing what Goffman (1964) refers to as a "spoiled identity".

I can think of at least three nurses who share a way of working/being which is
enabling and encouraging. They all meet people where they are and give out a lot
of positive energy which promotes self-esteem and self-confidence, which serves
to increase self-worth. In Phil's practice in particular, everything is "interesting"
rather than "good or bad"'.

This final premise, despite its apparent simplicity, may well be the most
provocative. Psychiatric nursing, which for so long has been embedded
within the medical establishment, often has found itself caught up in the
'power play' of psychiatry. Psychiatric nurses often find themselves cast
primarily in the role of custodians, managers and modifiers of the people
called 'patients' (cf. Whitehill, 1996). Many nurses might even be viewed as
having volunteered for such roles, finding it less demanding, on a human
level, to play them, than to relate to 'persons' and their personal distress.
The 'retreat' of psychiatric nurses into the role of therapist, of whatever
persuasion, might even be viewed as further evidence of nurses' difficulty
in dealing with the basic challenge of 'nursing' people in mental distress
(Michael, 1994). The final premise implies a need for nurses to make their
own contribution to the deconstruction of mental illness, and to the
development of a method of practice which might reflect the 'working in
partnership' enshrined in the political rhetoric of nursing policy (Department of Health, 1994). Such a method might also require nurses to reflect
better the fact that the experience of being in mental distress derives from
the real world of social and interpersonal relationships. It is there, rather
than in the artificial construction of 'mentalism' and its associated diagnostic states, that nursing practice might find its proper focus.

Summary

This chapter has provided a sketch of the territory of psychiatric nursing,
viewed by a recipient of nursing and a provider. By drawing on our
separate and mutual experiences we have attempted to offer a view of

psychiatric nursing grounded in our reflections on the process of caring. The four premises which anchor this perspective, and which derive from the work of a larger group of nurse practitioners, serve as introductions to a theory of psychiatric nursing; one which might more appropriately reflect the practical issues involved in giving and receiving care.

References

Barker, P. (1989) Reflections on the philosophy of psychiatric nursing. *Journal of Advanced Nursing* **26** (2) 131–141.

Barker, P. (1995) Promoting growth through community mental health nursing. *Mental Health Nursing* **15** (3), 12–15.

Barker, P. & Stevenson, C. (1996) Collaborative caring in psychiatric nursing. Unpublished manuscript, University of Newcastle Upon Tyne, Newcastle Upon Tyne.

Barker, P., Reynolds, W. & Ward, T. (1995a) The proper focus of nursing: a critique of the 'caring' ideology. *International Journal of Nursing Studies* **32** (4), 386–397.

Barker, P., Stevenson, C., Conway, E. *et al.* (1995b) *Toward a Theory of Psychiatric Nursing Practice: The Tyneside View.* The University of Newcastle Upon Tyne, Newcastle Upon Tyne.

Bauer, B. & Hull, S.S. (1986) *Essentials of Health Care Planning and Intervention.* H.B. Saunders, Philadelphia.

Department of Health (1994) *Working in Partnership.* HMSO, London.

Goffman, E. (1964) *Stigma: Notes on the Management of Spoiled Identity.* Penguin, Harmondsworth.

Gournay, K. (1995) Mental health nurses working purposefully with people with serious and enduring mental illness – an international perspective. *International Journal of Nursing Studies* **32** (4), 341–352.

King, S. (1991) *Needful Things.* Hodder & Stoughton, London.

Michael, S. (1994) Invisible skills: how recognition and value need to be given to the 'invisible skills' frequently used by mental health nurses, but often unrecognized by those unfamiliar with mental health nursing. *Journal of Psychiatric and Mental Health Nursing* **1** (1), 56–57.

Peplau, H.E. (1952) *Interpersonal Relations in Nursing: A Conceptual Frame of Reference for Psychodynamic Nursing.* Putnam, New York.

Porter, R. (1987) *A Social History of Madness.* Weidenfield and Nicholson, London.

Sullivan, H.S. (1953) *The Interpersonal Theory of Psychiatry.* WW Norton, New York.

Watson, O. (1968) *The Longman Dictionary.* Longman, London.

Watson, J. (1989) Watson's philosophy and theory of human caring. In *Conceptual Models for Nursing Practice* 3rd edn. (Riehl-Sisca J. ed.). Appelton and Lange, Norwalk, Connecticut, pp. 121–139.

Whitehill, I. (1996) General reflection. *Nursing Times* **92** (21), 61–62.

Wright, B. (1991) Labelling: the need for greater person-environment individuation. In *Handbook of Social and Clinical Psychology: The Health Perspective* (Snyder, C.R. & Forsyth, D.R. eds). Pergamon Press, Oxford, pp. 416–421.

3 Caring About the Client: The Role of Gender, Empathy and Power in the Therapeutic Process

Ruth Gallop

'A way of being in the world'

Many years ago as a student nurse, I was taken to the 'back' ward of a large psychiatric hospital. For 3 months, 2 days a week, I spent time on this ward, a ward full of chronic patients with minimal staff coverage. I was assigned to a 'difficult' patient. Like me, she was in her twenties. She had a diagnosis of schizophrenia but, more problematically, she rejected everyone in a most dis-engaging manner. She was considered a 'bad' patient. Needless to say, as a young, idealistic student, I saw her and the problems she presented as a challenge. Even then, though, part of me questioned the ethics of 'parachuting' in students with lots of time for patient interaction, who would then leave. However, I decided that perhaps I could, by attempting to connect with her, find a piece in her that other nurses would be attracted to. When I left she gave me a present she had made (hand-knitted woollen slippers). Although we were not permitted to accept gifts, I accepted the slippers, deciding that the wrath of my instructor was easier to endure than the injury I would inflict by refusing her gift. I gave her a card telling her how much I had gained from the opportunity of knowing and working with her.

Thus I was hooked into the themes that have since driven my professional career both as a clinician and as a researcher: understanding the therapeutic relationship or interpersonal process (later this was to crystallise into efforts to understand empathy); working with clients perceived as 'difficult'; and working with women.

Despite the overall discursive nature of this chapter, I have found it necessary to insert a narrative voice for the explication of the themes and the linkages between the themes. In reality, the integrity of the argument outlined later in this chapter requires the insertion of the narrative. My thinking about the essential qualities of the psychiatric/mental health nursing role has been influenced by the experience of being a woman, being a nurse and living and working in North America. In a sense, the combining of the discursive and narrative voices represents an attempt to capture a personal and professional journey of understanding: an attempt to capture the evolution of my intellectual and intuitive understanding of the heart of psychiatric nursing. Like a fugue, these two voices are inter-twined and inseparable.

In the text PMHN may refer to the 'psychiatric/mental health nurse' or to 'psychiatric/mental health nursing', as defined by context. The term PMHN reflects the reality that a nurse may work with clients with iden-tified disorders and/or mental health problems. The term 'mental health nurse' is not used in North America. Commonly, nurses within this area of speciality are called psychiatric nurses but I prefer a phrase that reflects the broader context of the field.

My early nursing career took me to a leading psychoanalytical hospital where I began to encounter young female patients with diagnoses which would later be subsumed under the rubric of borderline personality dis-order (BPD). Bright, articulate and troubled women, they challenged and tested staff, alternately adoring and reviling them. By the mid-1970s, after working in the USA and England, I was Associate Director of an inpatient facility specialising in the long-term treatment of BPD patients. (For 'patients' read 'women': although it is stated that distribution of this diagnostic category is not gender-specific, over 70% of persons hospitalised with the diagnosis of BPD in North America are female (Herman & van der Kolk, 1987), and I can't recall seeing a male hospitalised with the diagnosis of BPD.)

I was familiar with the work of Thomas Main and his seminal article 'The ailment' (Main, 1962) based on work at the Cassell Hospital in Richmond, England; and James Masterson, author of *Treatment of the Borderline Ado-lescent* (Masterson, 1972), was a regular visiting professor for the unit. These authors aroused in me an interest in trying to understand the nature of the staff–patient relationship with patients who are perceived as diffi-cult.

In my subsequent academic and consulting career I have attempted to answer some of the questions raised in this clinical work. I have come to wonder about the interplay between the themes of interpersonal relation-ship, difficult patients, and women. These themes seem particularly rele-vant to some of the unique qualities that characterise the practice of psychiatric/mental health nursing. Over time my understanding of these themes has altered, modified and expanded. I still believe in the cen-trality of the interpersonal relationship but believe that many of the defining qualities of that relationship are shaped by gender: the parti-cular way empathy and/or caring develops in women, the role of the nurse/woman in the health care system, the social conditions of practice, and, more generally, the social condition of women in society. I believe that nurses have the potential to have relationships with clients which may be qualitatively different from clients' relationships with workers in other disciplines. I also believe that whether a nurse achieves his/her potential may depend on education, gender or history, or all three influences.

First, a number of caveats. Attempting to write about the relationship as the heart and soul of psychiatric/mental health nursing (PMHN) has not been easy. Certainly every psychiatric nursing text confirms the centrality of the nurse–patient relationship. Chapter after chapter details the importance of the relationship, describing the therapeutic use of self and the negative consequences when we fail to attend to the subjective experience of our patients. But how do I reconcile this espoused valuing of empathy and attention to the subjective experience of the other, with what I have observed in practice and in my own and others' research: nurses' failure to inquire and to attend; and their preference for carrying out administrative tasks, for giving advice rather than listening (Clark, 1981; Gallop *et al.*, 1989; Burcher, 1992). If I say that nurses (i.e. women) have acquired a capacity for connection more finely attuned than the capacity I find in many men, how do I reconcile this with my observation that many nurses seem not to care or listen, perhaps for reasons of individual history, systemic oppression or benign neglect? The constant dialectic of each situation, each assumption, each supposition, threatens to paralyse my attempts to write.

What I have written speaks to what I believe is the potential for psychiatric nursing. However, a number of aspects of the current situation in which nurses work, e.g. the dominance of the medical model, hierarchical organisation, devaluation of 'women's' work, inadequate educational opportunities, and the enormous pressures to find the cheapest generic worker, mean that nurses will have to struggle hard to achieve, let alone maintain, quality practice. Yet again, another dialectic rears its ugly head. I am not prepared to offer up the 'nurse (woman) as victim' (silenced and oppressed) as an explanatory model for our problems. Passivity will not advance our cause. I am aware that I write from a position of privilege – born into a middle-class family, well-educated and professionally successful. I recognise that many of my so-called successes depended initially on the assistance and 'permission' (benevolence) of another person, usually male with more power in the system; so on go the dilemmas. With these major caveats constantly in my mind, and hopefully in the mind of readers, I shall proceed.

The argument to be developed

In this chapter I will suggest that the potential power of psychiatric nursing comes from the unique nature of the caring relationship. The nature of this relationship, framed in notions of empathy, nurturing, connectiveness or intimacy (the specific word is problematic), derives not only from our professional role but also from our gender (whether as a consequence of social construction or biology is open for debate). Consequently, nursing may be a female profession rather than a profession with significant numbers of women. Further, I will consider whether the nature of the relationship, which I consider to be qualitatively different from the doctor-client relationship, functions under different power rules which alter the quality of and define the limits of the relationship ('power' here indicating boundary rules and obligations reflected in the power balance between client and health professional). Before doing so, it is necessary first to describe psychiatry in North America and the impact this model of psychiatry has had on nursing.

The dominant paradigm

In North America, the dominant paradigm for psychiatry is the medical model. The psychiatrist is the expert and all other disciplines serve to complement this expertise. The role of the psychiatrist is to diagnose and treat according to the specific 'disease' identified. These diseases are defined in the *Diagnostic and Statistical Manual* (DSM) of Mental Disorders of the American Psychiatric Association. The DSM, now in its fourth edition, was designed to provide systematic and reliable guidance on diagnosis. DSM diagnoses are based, with few exceptions, on behavioural signs and symptoms. Multi-dimensional determinants of disease are paid scant attention in the diagnostic labelling process. The DSM has become so central to the practice of psychiatry that psychiatric/mental health nursing is diagnosis-driven both in the framework offered for understanding the person who is a patient, and in directing intervention.

The corollary of this is that PMHN practice remains restricted to a limited paradigm in which diagnosis is the defining explanatory model. Research and/or clinical activity which attempts to look across diagnostic categories for common elements is discouraged. Until recently, research that considered the impact of contextual variables on the aetiology and expression of illness was limited. I say this, in spite of efforts by many nurses to broaden this paradigm. The *Canadian Standards of Psychiatric and Mental Health Nursing Practice* (Standards Committee of the Canadian Federation of Mental Health Nurses, 1995) were designed to provide a basis for the evaluation of nursing practice in any setting in which the promotion of mental health and/or the psychiatric care of the client is the focus. These Standards state 'the PMH nurse is particularly concerned with fostering the functional status of clients. The PMH nurse understands how the disease process, the recuperative powers and the level of mental health are affected by contextual factors' (Standards Committee of the Canadian Federation of Mental Health Nurses, 1995).

The influence of the medical model of psychiatry is enhanced by an increasing emphasis on the biological determinants of mental illness. The American Psychiatric Association designated the 1990s 'the Decade of the Brain'. Biological determinism as an explanatory model for all mental disorders diminishes the role of the individual, the family and the context, and raises the fantasy of a 'magic pill' for all that ails you. Hence the overuse of Prozac in America. No one would argue about the importance of understanding physiological/biological determinants of illness. However, biological determinism as a model of mental illness may be too reductionist. Helping the client who is depressed, is experiencing a thought disorder or has an eating disorder, requires more than the 'right' medication. Understanding the experiences of the individual requires careful attention to how the world and the people in an individual's world impact on all aspects of that individual.

The need to understand contextual variables is most clearly seen when considering the role of childhood abuse (physical, sexual, psychological) in the aetiology and expression of illness. Given the strong associations between a history of abuse and many psychiatric disorders, particularly in women, authors have increasingly challenged the 'pathologising' of abuse and have suggested that the absence of the ability to trust people, establish relationships, and have a strong sense of self is nothing more than a normal response to the betrayal of the abused person's childhood (Kroll, 1993). To shift the current medical model paradigm or even to fight for an expanded paradigm requires courage and understanding. It requires serious attention to the social context of mental health. A paradigm shift would be reflected in the practising PMHN's behaviour with clients, families and the health care team, as well as in research and the content of curricula.

Nursing, gender and empathy

Nursing and gender issues are inseparable in North America. In Canada over 96% of all RNs are female. In the province where I work, the number is almost 98%. Within psychiatric mental health nursing, the number of male nurses is slightly higher. In Ontario, 10% of registered nurses working in psychiatric/mental health nursing are male. This last number is possibly inflated by the number of male security staff in forensic settings where job security depends on obtaining nursing qualifications; where, in other words, nursing was not a deliberate career choice. In Canada generally, the vast majority of nurses are generalists, having a basic education in all major fields of nursing. In Western Canada, there are registered psychiatric nurses (RPN) prepared only for mental health practice (and ineligible for registration elsewhere in Canada). The Western Canadian model is comparable to the British educational model for mental health nurses.

In the United States all nursing education is based on the generalist model, with speciality education occurring at the post-basic level. The situation in Canada, where the number of males in nursing has not changed for many years despite vigorous efforts to recruit males, contrasts with that in many countries (e.g. Holland and Australia, which have higher percentages of males in nursing). The postulated explanations for the lack of males include: low status; sexism in faculties of nursing; nursing as women's work; and availability of higher education and alternative career choices. Regardless of the explanation, the consequence is that in Canada and the United States, nursing must be considered at the least a female-dominated profession and more likely a female profession. Just as fighter pilots are probably members of a male profession in which females may participate, nursing is a female profession in which males may participate. Given this, issues of gender and its implications for practice, particularly in a domain such a PMHN, cannot be ignored.

The therapeutic relationship

In PMHN the therapeutic relationship is the nurse's primary intervention. What is it that PMHNs do that makes them different from other professionals?

For a number of years I have taught a course on the theories of interpersonal process. In the course outline, I argue that an individual nurse's particular theoretical frame (nursing theory, cognitive-behavioural theory, psychodynamic theory) is imposed over and above certain pre-determined qualities of the patient/client–therapist relationship that reflect the therapist's 'way of being in the world'. These relationship qualities are a consequence of biology, culture and an evolving personal history; each of which is greatly influenced by gender. Initially the course was grounded in the work of early object-relations theorists such as Melanie Klein, Fairbairn and Margaret Mahler. Object-relations theory builds on the observation that individuals live simultaneously in internal and external worlds of real relationships and internal images that mix and mingle (Greenberg & Mitchell, 1983). Early theorists saw developmental tasks largely in terms of the person separating and individuating (Mahler, 1967, 1972), and did not consider gender difference or gender development. Fairbairn (1986), though, does describe the need for the therapist to demonstrate 'feminine' qualities in the psychotherapy of clients who have profound attachment difficulties.

However, over the years the course has concentrated increasingly on the works of Winnicott and more contemporary female authors such as Janet Sayers (1991), Jessica Benjamin (1988), Chodorow (1978; 1989), Gilligan (1982), and Jordan *et al.* (1991). These writers have challenged the traditional theory that 'normal' human development entails separation, 'a process of separating oneself out from the matrix of others' (Miller, 1991, p. 11). Also rejected is a corollary of that theory, that women are deficient, i.e. not as successful as men in achieving the outcomes of separation and autonomy, since women seem to place the highest priority on the integrity of relationships. In its place, these writers offer alternative models of women's psychological development based on a relationship perspective.

According to Chodorow, 'as a result of being parented primarily by a woman, men and women develop differently constructed selves' (1989, p. 184). From earliest childhood boys and girls are socialised differently: the qualities of caring/nurturing are nourished in females and may be selectively discouraged in males (Jordan *et al.*, 1991). While mothers are attuned to the internal states of the infant, male or female, young girls are socialised to attend to the affective states of others. Boys are encouraged to individuate, become separate, limit the primary identification with the mother. In general, the connection between a mother and her daughter is more sustained, partly due to identification with sameness and partly due to societal norms. Affective sensitivity and attunement to how others feel is encouraged more in girls, reflecting the mother–daughter connection, and this allows the daughter to feel more attached and understood.

Thus development takes place in the context of relationships. As Surrey (1991, p. 37) suggests, 'for women at all life stages, relational needs are primary and ... healthy, dynamic relationships are the motivating force that propels psychological growth'. Nurturing, caretaking, caring for and attending to others are practices that mothers teach their daughters, which become an instrinsic part of a woman's self in relation to others. The female sense of self is constructed around a sense of connection to the world. Men, on the other hand, develop a sense of self that is based more on denial of relationship, and a sense of the self as separate (Chodorow, 1989). Gilligan (1982) suggests that women's sense of self centres on issues of responsibility for, care of and inclusion of others. If one accepts these notions, the implications for PMHN in North America are profound.

The focus of psychiatric nursing and the development of empathy

As many authors have observed, nursing's early history is rooted deeply in nurturing. Women cared for the sick and injured of the family and community. As Peplau (1994) suggests, early psychiatric nursing pursued a nurturing role. Before the psychotropic medications of the late 1950s, psychiatric mental health nurses cared for, fed, bathed, applied wet packs to, and ensured the safety of, their clients. Peplau (1952) supplied a theoretical model for the therapeutic relationship, providing the impetus for emergent psychiatric nursing practice involving individual and group interventions. The centrality of the relationship has not altered.

If we agree that the focus of psychiatric nursing is still, as Peplau suggested, 'the problems of our patients', and that what we experience during interactions with clients determines what we do, then this suggests to me that we need to be experts in helping the client live the best possible life in an interpersonal world.

At the heart of these interventions, which are still the primary interventions of psychiatric mental health nursing, is the process of empathy, whereby the nurse comes to know and understand the world of the other and to use that understanding constructively. Psychiatric nurses are expected to help clients understand the impact of their mental illness or health problem and to help the clients contemplate choices and move to constructive changes. Empathy and the closely related construct 'intuition' require the capacity to attend to the feelings of another and to attend to the feelings of self in relation to the other. Empathy has been described as a 'cognitive-emotional fugue', highlighting the intertwining of cognitive and affective components of empathy (Lewis *et al.*, 1984). 'Therapeutic empathy' implies additionally the wish to know or experience the world of the other (Gallop *et al.*, 1990).

It is my contention that women are well positioned, because of their developmental histories, to use their relational skills to enhance their understanding of the client's experience. As women, psychiatric mental health nurses may be more attuned to the qualities of connectiveness or empathy that are hallmarks of female development. Even early object-relation theorists such as Fairbairn (1986) spoke of a 'feminine' function of psychotherapy that reflects the therapist's ability to be empathic or to be with the client. Empathy is not some mysterious quality which you either possess or not, 'it is learned [acquired] in relationships and over time in the course of relationships' (Kaplan, 1991).

While I argue that women, as a consequence of their social construction, have the opportunity for more developed empathy, empathy is not exclusively the domain of women. The capacity for empathy can be developed and enhanced in anyone but it cannot be taught in a traditional pedagogical manner. Empathy must be experienced, identified and reflected upon. Curricula and clinical supervision that espouse sharing of experiences, reflection and exploration of process phenomena as opposed to theories of communication or interpretive formulations may enhance empathy. Not surprisingly, research on the acquisition of empathy showed that the greatest sustained change occurred in situations that promoted reflection, i.e. groups in which students spoke about and reflected on feelings they had experienced, in a non-evaluative atmosphere facilitated by a leader whose own style was reflective (Sellick, 1991).

Unfortunately, opportunities for truly reflective experiences are uncommon in the many nursing programmes which promote acquisition of a pseudo-empathic style reflecting how an instructor or student thinks the student should or should not feel/think/behave. Of course, the first requirement in providing an appropriate educational experience is an educator who has the capacities for reflection and empathy. This clearly raises the question of how to educate the educators. For mental health teaching, an instructor's capacity to think (however creatively) is not sufficient. The necessary capacities to feel and reflect therapeutically are often only acquired through experience of formally established opportunities for self-reflection, on an individual or group therapy basis. Acquiring insight into how one's own personal baggage informs the way one is in the world helps a person know when and where she/he ends and the other begins. But most importantly, by experiencing an increased understanding of self and the difficulties of the human condition, one is better positioned to hear and reflect upon the human condition of others (i.e. be empathic).

Incongruities in practice: empathy, connectiveness, and gender

Some of the incongruities I have seen in the practice of the psychiatric mental health nurse can be understood by considering the role of empathy and connectiveness in the relational world of women. For years I have talked about problems which occur in team meetings; in particular, why nurses' voices have been unheard or silenced. Mohr (1995, p. 88) describes the myth of the multi-disciplinary team meeting (MDTM): 'a pleasing myth is that the MDTM is an exercise in egalitarianism and democratic principles'. In reality, the MDTM is strictly hierarchial, led by the psychiatrist-expert and directed at assessing the patient's progress as described in the DSM diagnosis and treatment protocol. Input by other disciplines is relevant to the extent that it reinforces or illuminates aspects of the 'scientific' model.

It is often apparent that physicians and nurses speak different languages in these meetings. The medical staff (either male or women educated in the male model) speak the language of science: objective; positivist; signs, symptoms, diagnoses; the language of 'authority'. Nurses speak the language of women: relationships; feelings; context and process. The consequence of this difference in language and facade of collaboration is that the nurse is both unheard and silenced. Initially, she is unheard: she speaks and her words fall onto deaf ears. Eventually, she is silenced, as the ignoring of her words makes explicit that what she has to say is of no consequence (unless it confirms the scientific). Her comments about process, context and relationships do little to illuminate presciptive indicators such as: Are the drugs working? Are the symptoms abating?

At one point in my career, I thought the answer was to teach nurses to speak like doctors, but I've changed my mind. The goal must be to find a way for importance to be attached to relational and affective issues. This is a daunting task in a time of financial restraint. But for our clients, the ability to live and participate in an interpersonal world, a world grounded in relationships, is central. When I asked clients/abuse survivors who were helping me prepare a questionnaire for nursing staff what they most wanted from nursing staff, they said 'empathy' (they did not know that I do research on empathy).

Perspectives on 'difficult' patients

Recognising that for women relationships and self in relation to others are central, helps me understand the finding in our research that nurses and physicians had different explanatory models for perceptions of difficult patients. Nurses and doctors perceived the same patients as difficult. However, nurses (women) explained their perception of these patients as 'difficult' in terms of failed relationships in the patients' lives, and the nurses' own failure to establish a therapeutic relationship, or do more for the patients. Physicians (men) explained difficulty in terms of the patient's failure to respond to medication or the patient being not ready to use the help the physician had to offer (Gallop & Wynn, 1987; Gallop *et al.* 1993). In recent research concerning the limits of the nurse–client relationship, nurses state that clients talk differently to nurses and physicians 'because we are women, because we have less authority' (Gallop *et al.*, 1996).

Caring about clients

Psychiatric mental health nurses should start discussing ways to demonstrate that actively 'caring about' clients is both appropriate and therapeutic. 'Caring about' does not mean personal disclosure or over-involvement but it does mean acknowledging the importance of relationships in women's lives and of being real in the relationship. It of course requires theoretical knowledge, so that the understanding acquired by empathy and 'caring about' the client can be used to facilitate growth. It is important to recognise that professional caring or caring-as-work is different from maternal caring. According to Stiver (1991) objectivity and distancing play a key role in current models of therapeutic relationships. Therapists are warned against being too involved, caring too much, being too available.

The characteristics of objectivity and distance are consistent with a masculine model of separation and detachment and may be a defence against qualities of warmth, connection, interest and 'caring about' the client. This is not to suggest that the qualities of empathy, warmth, or being real in the relationship are the domains solely of women, but rather that these qualities are considered female qualities. Benjamin (1994) suggests that the need to defend against these qualities stems from men's fear of the power of the primary mother–infant relationship and the lifelong struggle not to be dominated ever again. The qualities of warmth, empathy and realness are qualities identified over and again by clients as those qualities missing in the current mental health care system (Church, 1992; Stiver, 1991).

In a revealing paper, Guntrip (1975) describes his own psychoanalysis with Winnicott and contrasts it to an earlier analysis. He saw Winnicott in the transference as the ultimate good mother, valuing the child, allowing attachment and demonstrating caring. These 'feminine' qualities facilitated Guntrip's own ability to feel alive, creative and cared about. This analysis contrasted starkly with the cool, detached, masculine style of his previous analysis.

Illustration

These issues can be illustrated further by considering the female client with a borderline personality disorder (BPD). This group of clients is predominately female and is defined by a set of characteristics many of which pertain to relational issues (unstable, intense relationships; frantic efforts to avoid real or imagined abandonment). Generally clients with this diagnosis are viewed in a pejorative way. Clients are seen as manipulative, angry, seductive and difficult. The literature focuses on counter-transference issues centred on the risks of staff being exploited, over-involved, enmeshed and manipulated. The psychodynamic model of understanding of this disorder centres on the client's failure to separate and individuate from the mother (Masterson, 1972). A simple example will illustrate the potential role for empathy and caring about the client.

Jane, a 23-year-old client with a diagnosis of BPD is upset that she cannot go home for the weekend following a serious overdose. She turns on the nurses and starts screaming: 'Nobody here cares about me'.

Nurses may have many differing reactions to Jane. But based on the admonition that being too concerned or too involved will support regression, any of the following responses may occur. One nurse may think 'You're right, I don't care' and say nothing; another may explain her role, 'Nurses are here to care – it is part of our job'; another nurse may provide a pseudo-empathic response, 'We all care about you'; yet another may interpret, 'Jane I think you are angry about not going home'; and another may be concerned that being empathic or sympathetic will increase Jane's potential for regression and respond by contradiction, 'You know that's not true'. Most likely Jane will be enraged by any of these responses and start escalating her behaviour.

A paradigm focused on empathy speaks to the subjective experience of the person and the affective component of the experience. Jane's subjective experience is one of 'not feeling cared about'; the affective component includes the feeling that being uncared for is unpleasant or distressing. An empathic response incorporates these dimensions; for example, 'it must feel awful to feel no one cares for you'.

Clearly Jane is not a child, but parallels to the child in distress are apparent. A mother must find ways to re-connect with her angry/distressed child. Nothing constructive can happen until the mother and child are re-engaged. Threats, physical punishment or abandonment may stop the behaviour but will not resolve the affect. The mother must shift from being the 'bad' mother to a 'caring' mother. Similarly the nurse must be perceived as caring. Being concerned does not mean that the nurse rewards, condones or is manipulated by the behaviour. Instead the nurse understands the distress, cares about how awful Jane is feeling, and recognises the feelings of 'aloneness' experienced by a woman in a world where self-in-relation-to-others is the defining characteristic of her persona. Unfortunately, existing paradigms of treatment for BPD have promoted the notion that clinicians need to be watchful and alert for manipulation and exploitation. The image of the patient as 'bad' or 'devious' devalues the distress of the client (Gallop, 1985). While it is indeed important to reflect on one's involvement and to receive adequate supervision with these very difficult clients, caring about the client should be permitted, and indeed encouraged.

Adler (1992) has written extensively on the difficulties of establishing a therapeutic alliance with the client with a BPD. Many of these clients seem to share histories in which they experience not feeling cared about and many have been abused (physically, psychologically and/or sexually). Briere (1992) and Kroll (1993) point out there is a strong concordance between the characteristics of the BPD and the consequences of childhood abuse. The life experiences of people with BPD have not provided opportunities for the internalisation of a strong sense of self, nor for a capacity for sustaining positive images. According to Adler (1992, p. 252), the client has 'lost the ability to remember the therapist [nurse] with *feeling* as someone who cares, soothes, or holds'. Hence, for the nurse each new contact provides an opportunity for the client to experience connection and engagement, however transient. The nurse is well positioned to hear the client and to help the client make sense of his/her history by demystifying and normalising experience. It should not be surprising to a nurse that a client with a history of childhood abuse has difficulty trusting or believing people. This is a 'normal' response to the betrayal of childhood and the empathic nurse can help the client recognise this 'normalcy'. Consequently, the treatment goal for the client with BPD may be to connect and individuate rather than to separate and individuate.

Empowerment of nurses: on being heard

Ironically, the unheard voice of the client with a BPD may not be so different from the nurse's experience of being unheard. Nurses must acknowledge and act upon the opportunities to enact power in a different voice. While I would not want to overdraw parallels between the dilemmas of the client with a BPD and the nurses working in a system where their voices are often unheard or unattended, nurses are at risk of acting out their own experience of being 'dominated' by the system and of telling the client what to do, think, or control.

Although I am still intrigued with the micro-process, attention to social context requires consideration of 'macro' societal forces. In a country where 96% of the nurses are female, nursing must take on the mantle of being not only a female profession but also a feminist profession. Being a feminist has little to do with how you dress, whether or not you use make-up, or whether you are a Marxist, but a whole lot to do with recognising that we live and work in a male-dominated culture in which male-oriented theories of psychological development and normalcy have shaped contemporary thinking. It has to do with recognising that women's voices have been silenced (both our voices and our female clients' voices), their stories disregarded, and their work often undervalued. We need to understand the linkages between being a woman/daughter, sister, mother, and being a nurse. Are these permeable boundaries?

Nurses can learn most, not from the models of domination, or of sanctioned, legal or expert power, but rather from considering the importance of the nurse–patient relationship and the role of interpersonal intimacy or caring, in the light of feminist or emancipatory goals such as choice, awareness, freedom to act intentionally, and involvement in change. Nurses espouse valuing and attending to the subjective experience of the other, of understanding the 'lived experience' of the other. All of these values are completely compatible with feminist goals, which reflect the feminine relationship.

If PMHN is to move towards identifying emancipatory or feminist outcomes as valid nursing outcomes then we need to understand by what means we achieve them. If the nursing care we provide has some of the qualities of care I listed earlier then we need to understand the potential and limitations of these qualities in shaping nurses' work. What if PMHN practice is a practice that can utilise effectively certain qualities which have been traditionally identified as female? Does this present a problem? Not if we embrace these qualities and acknowledge the difference they can make. As women we are well positioned to recognise that the social reality of many women's lives involves abuse, economic hardship and unfulfilled aspirations. We also need to recognise that the PMHN has colluded with the psychological models of normalcy that focus on independence, separation and power as the ultimate expressions of success and sound mental health.

PMHN as women must recognise that they share many of the problems of their female clients and that if they do not recognise and challenge their own powerlessness in the system then they will be ill-equipped to help others. Roberts (1983) spoke of nurses as members of an oppressed group. She described the process whereby senior nurses identify with the oppressor (i.e. ally with physicians and administrators) in order to have 'power-over' front-line clinicians. It is often all too easy for exceptional psychiatric nurses to be seduced by the 'power-over' model, whereby a senior person (often physician) 'allows' a nurse to run a group, become a therapist, or participate in research – a 'privilege' which can easily be withdrawn.

Personal empowerment or 'power-to' lies at the heart of feminist empowerment (Kitzinger, 1991). Personal empowerment involves a sense of control over one's own thoughts, feelings and behaviours, in contrast to 'power-over' involving control of others (Yoder & Kahn, 1992). Feminist therapy focuses on facilitating the empowerment of others. Providing the 'power-to' or sense of personal empowerment is consistent with the empathic role of the PMHN. At the micro-level, attending to, valuing, and taking seriously the experience of the other is in itself empowering. For the abused client, having her abuse believed by the nurse is empowering. Having her telling of abuse silenced or seen as a ploy for attention is disempowering. Feminist methods focus on hearing the story of the other (attending to the subjective experience) not only in a purely intellectual, information gathering mode, but also in order to formulate and diagnose. The aim instead is to listen in order to truly understand the meaning for the individual, the core requirement of empathy. This is the way for the PMHN to be in the world. The dilemma, of course, is that for PMHNs to take on this role in a way that is valued and acknowledged within the mental health domain requires that psychiatric/mental health nursing undergoes fundamental social change – it must itself feel empowered with the power to change and to create a collective voice. Addressing the problem of how a disempowered profession creates a supportive empowering environment, in which we can advance both client and professional interests, is one of the major challenges facing the profession.

References

Adler, G. (1992) The myth of the therapeutic alliance with borderline patients revisited. In *Handbook of Borderline Disorders* (D. Silve & M. Rosenbluth eds). International Universities Press, Madison, Connecticut, pp. 251–265.

Benjamin, J. (1988) The first bond. In *The Bonds of Love*. Pantheon Books, New York, pp. 11–50.

Benjamin, J. (1994) The omnipotent mother: a psychoanalytic study of fantasy and reality. In *Representations of Motherhood* (Bassin, D., Honey, M. & Kaplan, M.M. eds.). Yale University Press, New Haven, Connecticut, pp. 129–146.

Briere, J. (1992) *Child Abuse Trauma: Theory and Treatment of the Lasting Effects*. Sage, Newbury Park, California.

Burcher, E. (1992) The investigation of public health nurses' inquiry into the subjective experience of new mothers prior to giving advice. Unpublished Master's thesis, University of Toronto, Toronto.

Chodorow, N. (1978) *The Reproduction of Mothering: Psychoanalysis and the Sociology of Gender*. University of California Press, Berkeley, California.

Chodorow, N. (1989) *Feminism and Psychoanalytic Theory*. Yale University Press, New Haven, Connecticut.

Church, K. (1992) *Moving Over: A Commentary on Power-Sharing. Psychiatric Survivor Leadership Facilitation Program*. The Ontario Ministry of Health Community Mental Health Branch, Toronto.

Clark, J. (1981) Communication in nursing. *Nursing Times*, January, 12–18.

Fairbairn, W. (1986) A revised psychopathology of the psychoses and psychoneuroses. In *Essential Papers on Object Relations* (P. Buckley ed.). New York University Press, New York, pp. 71–101.

Gallop, R. (1985) The patient is splitting: everyone knows and nothing happens. *Journal of Psychosocial Nursing* 23 (4), 6–10.

Gallop, R. & Wynn, F. (1987) The difficult in-patient: identification and response by staff. *Canadian Journal of Psychiatry* 32, 211–215.

Gallop, R., Lancee, W. & Garfinkel, P. (1989) How nurses respond to the label 'borderline personality disorder'. *Hospital and Community Psychiatry* 40, 815–819.

Gallop, R., Lancee, W. & Garfinkel, P. (1990). The empathic process and its mediators: a heuristic model. *The Journal of Nervous and Mental Disease* 178, 649–654.

Gallop, R., Lancee, W. & Shugar, G. (1993) Residents' and nurses' perceptions of difficult-to-treat short stay patients. *Hospital and Community Psychiatry* 44, 352–357.

Gallop, R., Donner, G., Kasta, W. & Lancee, W. (1996) *The Nature and Limits of the Professional Role. Final Report, Quality of Nurse Worklife*. Research Unit, University of Toronto, Toronto.

Gilligan, C. (1982) *In a Different Voice*. Harvard University Press, Cambridge, Massachusetts.

Greenberg, J.R. & Mitchell, S.A. (1983) *Object Relations and Psychoanalytic Theory*. Harvard University Press, Cambridge, Massachusetts.

Guntrip, H. (1975) My experience of analysis with Fairbairn and Winnicott. In *Essential Papers in Object-Relations* (P. Buckley ed.). New York Universiry Press, New York, pp. 450–468.

Herman, J. & van der Kolk, B. (1987) Traumatic antecedents of borderline personality disorder. In *Psychological Trauma* (B.A. van der Kolk ed.). American Psychiatric Press, Washington, District of Columbia, pp. 111–126.

Jordan, J., Kaplan, A., Miller, J.B., Stiver, I. & Surrey, J. (1991) *Women's Growth in Connection: Writings from the Stone Center*. Guilford Press, New York.

Kaplan, A. (1991) Empathic communication in the psychotherapy relationship. In *Women's Growth in Connection: Writings from the Stone Center* (J.V. Jordan, A.G. Kaplan, J.B. Miller, I.P. Stiver & J.L. Surrey eds). Guilford Press, New York, pp. 44–50.

Kitzinger, C. (1991) Feminism, psychology and the paradox of power. *Feminism and Psychology* **1**, 111–129.

Kroll, J. (1993) *PTSD/Borderlines in Therapy: Finding the Balance*. W.W. Norton, New York.

Lewis, M., Sullivan, M. & Michaelson, L. (1984) The cognitive-emotional fugue. In *Emotions, Cognitions and Behavior* (C. Izzard, J. Kagan & R. Zajonc eds). Cambridge University Press, Cambridge, pp. 264–288.

Mahler, M. (1967) On human symbiosis and the vicissitudes of individuation. *Journal of the American Psychoanalytic Association* **15**, 740–763.

Mahler, M. (1972) On the first three subphases of the separation-individuation process. *International Journal of Psychoanalysis* **53**, 333–338.

Main, T. (1962) The ailment. Reprinted in *The Essential Papers on Object Relations* (P. Buckley ed.). New York University Press, New York, 1986, p. 419–446.

Masterson, J. (1972) *Treatment of the Borderline Adolescent*. Brunner/Mazel, New York.

Miller, J.B. (1991) The development of women's sense of self. In *Women's Growth in Connection: Writings from the Stone Center* (J.V. Jordan, A.G. Kaplan, J.B. Miller, I.P. Stiver & J.L. Surrey eds). Guilford Press, New York, pp. 11–26.

Mohr, W. (1995) A critical reappraisal of a social form in psychiatric care settings: the multidisciplinary team meeting as a paradigm case. *Archives in Psychiatric Nursing* **9**, 85–91.

Peplau, H. (1952) *Interpersonal Relations in Nursing*. G.P. Putnam and Sons, New York.

Peplau, H. (1994) Psychiatric mental health nursing: challenge and change. *Journal of Psychiatric and Mental Health Nursing* **1**, 3–7.

Roberts, S.J. (1983) Oppressed group behavior: implications for nursing. *Advances in Nursing Science* **5** (4), 21–30.

Sayers, J. (1991) *Mothering Psychoanalysis*. Penguin Books, Harmondsworth.

Sellick, K. (1991) Nurses' interpersonal behaviours and the development of helping skills. *International Journal of Nursing Studies* **28**, 3–11.

Standards Committee of the Canadian Federation of Mental Health Nurses (1995) *Canadian Standards of Psychiatric/Mental Health Nursing Practice*. Prepared by Standards Committee of the Canadian Federation of Mental Health Nurses, an interest group of the Canadian Nurses Association.

Stiver, I.P. (1991) The meaning of care: reframing treatment models. In *Women's Growth in Connection: Writings from the Stone Center* (J.V. Jordan, A.G. Kaplan, J.B. Miller, I.P. Stiver & J.L. Surrey eds). Guilford Press, New York, pp. 250–267.

Surrey, J. (1991) The self-in relation: a theory of women's development. In *Women's Growth in Connection: Writings from the Stone Center* (J.V. Jordan, A.G. Kaplan, J.B. Miller, I.P. Stiver, J.L. Surrey eds). Guilford Press, New York, pp. 51–66.

Yoder, J. & Kahn, A. (1992) Toward a feminist understanding of women and power. *Psychology of Women Quarterly* **16**, 381–388.

4 Coercion, Control and Mental Health Nursing

David Glenister

Introduction

The promotion of the primacy of caring in nursing (Benner & Wrubel, 1989) may soothe consciences and present a favourable image to others, yet at the same time deny the centrality of coercion and control in mental health nursing practice. Demonstrating a welcome frankness, earlier handbooks for the instruction of psychiatric nurses (e.g. Ackner, 1964) cautioned against the uncritical adoption of notions of 'care' by mental health nurses. The issues of coercion and control are managed in several ways within current mental health nursing literature. In textbooks for student mental health nurses, the therapeutic nature of nursing is often taken for granted, and the issue of social control is simply not addressed. In nursing policy, the duty of care is promoted, and the importance of respecting clients' choices is indicated, while the use of the euphemistic term 'care without consent' obscures coercion (UKCC, 1996, p. 20).

Another form of denial is found in historical studies. Nolan's (1993) history of mental nursing described the use of fear as a means of social control in earlier decades, without discussion of the extent to which this practice is evident today. Even when the relevance of the sociology of social control has been examined in relation to mental health nursing (for example, Symonds, 1991; Porter, 1993), nurses' and users' experiences of social control have rarely been examined.

In the author's opinion, both student mental health nurses, who are socialised into the use and abuse of power during their education, and service users are poorly served by an unwillingness to debate critically issues related to acts of coercion and control. An open debate might help prevent the excesses of violence and permissiveness that may physically and psychologically damage those involved. In the Orwellian present, the 'nursespeak' vocabulary substitutes 'care' for 'control', 'cooperation' for 'conflict', and 'mental health services' for 'psychiatric surveillance'. Critical debate about what mental health nurses do can only commence once the nursing vocabulary, which restricts the range and use of words, and therefore thinking and talking, is challenged.

In this chapter, the author explores violence, coercion and control in mental health services by drawing upon some forms of evidence often ignored by those who seek to understand the current state of mental health nursing; in particular, autobiography, governmental inquiries and reports. Nevertheless, these forms of evidence offer insights into mental health nursing practice. Autobiography can be seen as a form of ethnography in which people struggle to make sense of their experience. Official reports can be seen as case studies (Clarke, 1991), offering insights that may be generalisable to other settings. The Mental Health Act Commission's bi-annual reports are a rich source of data concerning the current state of mental health services. Managers' and academics' current enthusiasm for 'evidence based health care' elevates the status of research-based evidence, especially evidence arising from clinical trials, but may at the same time devalue these less systematic but still valid forms of evidence.

Today British student nurses often have no sense of being higher education students, because of the demands of their work placements, and no sense of being nurses, because of the academic demands made on them by higher education institutions. Student nurses learn and undertake actions, and hear and then espouse ideas through a process of assimilation. Acts that were viewed with horror or fear in the first few months, become part of mundane reality over time. So much jargon will be learned that the student will become almost unintelligible to the lay person. In the author's opinion, part of the trick of remaining human despite being a student nurse, lies in retaining a sense of strangeness and wonder, as if one were an anthropologist working with a largely unmodernised and remote tribe, and attending to what people do and the ideas and values that people use to justify what they do. Periodically ignoring the instructions and refusing the jargon of lecturers, nurse managers, and one's peers is one way the author has found of maintaining some semblance of personal integrity while working as a nurse. In this spirit, the author writes here in the third person, in order to attain a sense of disengagement from the familiar.

Violence

More than 40 years after Barton's (1959) assault upon British institutional psychiatry, and more than 10 years after Beardshaw's (1981) catalogue of mental health nursing brutality, Beardshaw, in an oral submission to the Inquiry into Ashworth Hospital (Blom-Cooper, 1992), expressed regret that the days of bullying of mental health service users, and intimidation of those nurses who spoke out, were not over. A service user, in another oral submission to the Inquiry, reflected upon nurses' moral authority.

'They just get a kick out of being over us with power. Some have no sense and are so young. If I didn't live here I wouldn't believe any decent person could treat another so bad. Patients are supposed to be sick but what is their excuse?'
(Blom-Cooper, 1992, p. 80)

The same question can be asked in relation to nurses working in other settings. In interviews concerning ethical dilemmas encountered by student nurses during their placements, Clarke (1994) noted the frequency with which students mentioned an almost total reliance upon medication, and 'piling in' to restrain a patient prior to seclusion or injection. Wallcraft and Reed (1992), in guidelines for mental health workers, described a potent combination of violence and denial in mental health nursing practice.

> 'On more than one occasion I was beaten up by nurses. They actually enjoyed doing it. And when they used to tell me that no one would believe me they were right. Like the charge nurse once said to me, "Who is going to believe anyone in a mental hospital ? We just put it down to you being ill. Tell people what you want, but they are not going to believe you".'
>
> (Bell, undated, cited in Wallcraft & Reed, 1992)

The evidence of the survivors of psychiatric services and the survivors of political torture indicates that their experiences are similar, in that both are told that no one will believe them (Lawrence, 1992a, 1992b).

Violence between users, and the fear of such violence, also exist. In a study of users' experience of psychiatric hospital wards (Lovell, 1995), 72% of users reported they had been frightened by other users, and 52% reported being threatened verbally or physically. In mixed-gender acute psychiatric hospital wards, 'women feel very frightened to sleep in dormitories or single rooms leading from corridors that are easily accessible to male patients' (HMSO, 1993). The Mental Health Act Commission (HMSO, 1993) reported 'a woman suffering from puerperal depression was admitted informally with her baby ... said she was nervous of venturing away from her room ... she spent long periods standing as a sentry at her door'. In this sense, admission into an inpatient psychiatric unit can be regarded as a form of trauma, which people recall with anxiety. At worst, violence and the fear of violence distort and deny any possibility of therapeutic relationships between nurses and users.

Violence appears to be an integral aspect of psychiatric services, which must be acknowledged, at some level, by both victim and perpetrator. For the victim, violence is usually a humiliating experience, worsened by shame and others' refusal to listen and understand. For the perpetrator, the act of violence may corrode self-respect. However, Barton (1976) indicated the limitation of blaming isolated individuals, or indeed, isolated institutions.

> 'Brutality, browbeating, rough handling, harshness, teasing and general illtreatment always lie latent in institutions, smouldering and ready to burst into flames at any time ... The presumption that such things do not or cannot happen has been shown again and again to be naive and fatuous.'
>
> (Barton 1976, p. 10–11)

The subsequent history of psychiatric services indicates that managerial supervision is not sufficient to ensure violence is eliminated. A more challenging view is that violence is inescapable in institutions associated with coercion and control.

Coercion

Coercion is defined here as the use of legitimated physical force to achieve submission. Coercion is legitimated by mental health legislation, which prescribes the circumstances in which coercion can be used; in contrast, violence is not legitimated by legislation. In mental health services coercion involves enforced admission and detention, the forcible administration of medications, seclusion, and control and restraint. Coercion also exists outside of institutions; for example, in neighbourhoods, where socially sanctioned coercion may involve harassment of unpopular individuals, when this is legitimated by popular opinion. Additionally, detaining and restraining are not unknown among family and friends. On the basis of cross-cultural comparisons, Horwitz (1982) suggested those groups and individuals who are marginal to the social order are more likely to be coerced. In Britain, black people and women appear to be more likely to be subjected to coercive interventions.

According to the Sixth Report of the Mental Health Act Commission (HMSO, 1995), psychiatric services are 'unwelcome, unsupportive and alien' to the culture and needs of the black population. Black people who come into contact with psychiatric services are more likely to be detained and treated using high doses of medication (HMSO, 1993), and more likely to be treated in secure settings. Black people in mental health services dominated by white people felt 'isolated, misunderstood, and discriminated against' (HMSO, 1995). The Report of Inquiry into the death of Orville Blackwood (Special Hospital Services Authority, 1993) suggested racist stereotypes were evident in decision-making about diagnosis and estimations of dangerousness. A 'Review of the Report of the Enquiry into the Care and Treatment of Christopher Clunis' based on a 'black perspective' (Harris, 1994) suggested that medical and nursing care was often 'colour-blind' and insensitive to cultural variation. Shepard's (1995) review of official inquiries, on behalf of the Zito Trust, suggested a consistent basic lack of awareness about racism and culture in mental health services. Coercion appears to be more readily applied to black people than to white people, and clinical decisions appear to be informed by racist stereotypes, possibly because of the marginal position of black people in the white social order.

In a course assignment, Barrett (1992), a third year student nurse, sought to identify with a woman who was subject to coercive interventions.

> 'A nineteen year old patient informs me that she is pregnant and will shortly give birth. Her evidence is an absence of periods for nine months, approximately the time she has been forced to submit to regular neuroleptic injections. Every two weeks she is routinely raped. Her jeans and underwear are pulled down. An ice cold penis penetrates her flesh shooting its thick oily load inside her ... 400 mg. The girl is traumatised, humiliated. The nurses stand smugly around her, willing to lend their weight to this therapeutic gang-bang.'
>
> (Barrett, 1992)

Barrett's storytelling and use of metaphor challenge the reader to imagine the routine violence of the enforced administration of medications, from the user's perspective. The significant number of male nurses who are disciplined for assaults upon female users (Department of Health, 1994), suggests that this intimation of sexual sadism may have some general validity.

Women's identity as strong, independent and autonomous persons is often undermined by male mental health workers who have stereotyped images of gender (Pollock & West, 1984). A psychologist who gave evidence to the Ashworth Hospital Inquiry stated:

'I have ... learnt that in order to survive a system, women will conform to it with the loss of any vitality. They will conform by turning their anger and frustration on each other, and this is at the instigation of staff who promote pets and top dogs. They will conform by fighting themselves and ultimately turning their anger on themselves by self-harming behaviour to a shocking degree. They will conform by becoming docile and dependent like children.'

(Potier, cited by Blom-Cooper, 1992, p. 230)

In this study, it is clear that conformity was maintained through the establishment and maintenance of a social hierarchy, which turned women's anger and frustration away from figures of authority and towards each other. The women then became dependent upon figures of authority to restrain them from harming themselves and each other. In this sense, violence and coercion can be described as strategies for ensuring institutional social order.

Control

Control is here defined as the use of verbal persuasion. In mental health services, social control includes threatening, commanding and arguing, as well as talking with avowedly therapeutic intentions. Control is as evident in correction of dysfunctional thoughts in cognitive therapy as it is in psychoanalytical interpretation. In post-war British society, there has been a slow, steady shift towards promoting the primacy of the individual in society, and a privatised therapeutic relationship within psychiatric services. Horwitz (1982) suggested that societies in which the individual has primacy over the group have treatments oriented to the individual's elaboration of meaning, and the promotion of individual autonomy within a privatised therapeutic relationship. In contrast, societies in which the group has primacy over the individual have treatments oriented to ritual expression, social conformity and collective participation.

Following Horwitz (1982), it can be suggested that the modernisation of psychiatric services has involved the loss of the traditional site of coercion, the hospital, and the extension of controlling services, for example, psychotherapy. The research of Main et al. (1991) and Lucksted and Coursey (1995) suggests that users are more aware of the power staff have to control patients than are the staff themselves. Furthermore, the impact of control should not be under-estimated.

'Some portion of the damage I feel I have sustained during the past twenty-five years in the psychiatric system has been due to padded cells, drug 'cocktails' and the prevalent use of the power to threaten. But a great part has been a result of psychiatry's refusal to give value to my personal perceptions and experience ... I cannot believe it is possible to dismiss as meaningless people's most vivid and challenging interior experiences and expect no harm to ensue.'

(Campbell, 1992, p. 122)

From the user's perspective, having control taken away appears to be one of the central features of mental health services. Chamberlin, a psychiatric service survivor, wrote:

'The whole experience of mental hospitalisation promotes weakness and dependency. Not only are the lives of the patients controlled, but patients are constantly told such control is for their own good, which they are unable to see because of their mental illness. Patients become unable to trust their own judgement, indecisive, overly submissive to authority, frightened of the outside world.'

(Chamberlin, 1988, p. 4)

From this perspective, survival of psychiatric services is the process of enduring devaluation, not just enduring violence and coercion. One of the central demands of some survivors of psychiatric services is for open acknowledgement of their experience.

'My world view and experience of living were unimportant. My distress was acknowledged only within a medical framework which I did not share. My differences in perception were dismissed as 'hallucinations'. The spiritual activity in my life has been written off as delusion. My difficulties around eating were pronounced a 'disorder'. The ways in which I expressed my distress or dissent were declared invalid, stupid or sick ... In some cultures I would have been seen as a gifted individual, but in Western culture my distress was medicalised in the exercise of social control.'

(Pembroke, 1991, p. 30)

Control, in this sense, circumscribes the limits of human experience and ensures that what passes for common sense is not challenged. The ability to define reality, and to have that reality accepted by others, is one definition of power. Evidence from service users, supported by evidence from official enquiries and reports, suggests that mental health services disempower by invalidating personal experiences.

However, control also involves directing attention away from issues that someone in distress might challenge. All too often people enter mental health services with practical problems – needs for decent housing, a job, and enough money to go on holiday – only to find themselves slotted into a therapeutic programme aimed at enhancing their insight or skills, which are deemed lacking. A wide range of issues are simply dismissed, for example economic and political problems, through being either ignored or interpreted away.

This is not to say there is no alternative to the control of users by nurses. Bloor *et al.* (1988) described residential workers in therapeutic communities who incited resident users to take control of the community. Cullen (1991) noted the manner in which behaviour therapists challenge users to take control and determine their own problems and targets. Barauch and Treacher (1978) noted how users sought to control others, including relatives and nurses, through adopting and utilising the low expectations contained within the sick role.

The social order of psychiatric services is more commonly maintained through control than coercion, and yet control is less dramatic and more difficult to identify and resist. Rather than disguising the struggle for control between users, nurses and doctors, and grudgingly acknowledging the supposed value of cooperation, there may be something to be said for an open (non-violent) conflict over control. Furthermore, recognising users' and nurses' power and their ability to control each other may be more mentally healthy for those involved since it recognises strength and determination.

Similarities between violence, coercion and social control

An examination of psychiatric services has indicated that nurses' use of violence, coercion and social control often involves denying the personal experiences and world views of users, and undermining users' trust in themselves and others. Nurses' use of violence, coercion and social control usually ensures the submission of users, thus ensuring the continuation of psychiatric social order, whether inside or outside the hospital. At this point, the author will now discuss the factors that contribute to the continuation of the psychiatric system, in particular psychodynamic, organisational and state factors.

The psychodynamics of coercion and control

Psychoanalytical research seeks to understand the influence of unconscious factors upon psychological and organisational order. Few attempts have been made to understand the nature of the impulses from which nurses defend themselves through work routines. Smith's (1986) action research study suggested that nurses have impulses towards violence, and Barrett (1992) has suggested the existence of impulses towards sexual sadism. The fear of psychic disintegration may be described as one of the most basic anxieties. Nurses also seek to defend themselves against impulses towards chaos.

'Our clients often openly reveal deep and apparently disturbing parts of themselves. These revelations of humanity may provoke contact with similar experiences in the nurses ... the lingering fear or nagging doubt that we may indeed be as mad or even madder than the patients fills the nurse with dread. The very idea of mental contamination has produced defences more effective than those found in barrier nursing.'

(Barrett, 1992)

A desire for self-preservation may result from nurses coercing and controlling because of fear. Clarke (1994) suggested that nurses were frightened of their own impulses towards chaos and destruction, and sought to be disciplined by those in authority in order to defend themselves against wayward impulses. By way of example, Cullen (1991) indicates the possibilities for extortion and harm in therapeutic practice and argues for the national and international regulation of practice. The regulation of nurses by statutory bodies, the standing of nursing leaders within staff organisations, and the enthusiasm of nurse managers may indicate a compulsion by nurses to be punished for their wayward impulses towards chaos and destruction.

Another mechanism is projective identification (Jureidini, 1990), in which the nurse does not perceive her own impulses and internal chaos, but rather identifies them as belonging to the user and attempts to control in that person the feelings that she cannot accept or recognise in herself. This mechanism may also express itself in controlling, coercive and violent behaviour. The nurse insists upon her caring nature and denies the extent to which she acts in a controlling, coercive or violent way, but readily accuses users of being manipulative, uncooperative or dangerous. To move beyond this mechanism might entail accepting that mental health nursing exists in a moral grey zone between caring and controlling.

The organisation of coercion and control

Bureaucracies are characterised by a clearcut hierarchy of authority, written rules and procedures, and full-time salaried officials. Their primary advantages are that they ensure decisions are not based upon whim, ensure a good level of competence amongst all staff, and discourage promotion through nepotism (Giddens, 1993). However, they suffer from a lack of flexibility and responsiveness. A good deal of nurses' energy is spent in attempting to establish satisfactory relationships with peers, and this is often more difficult than working with users. Hayes (1979) offered penetrating insights into some of these problems.

> 'One of the most striking characteristics of psychiatric nursing is its structure ... The positions which actually provide the service to the intended population are those closest to the bottom. Orders about the way the service is to be provided work their way from a superior to an inferior position. The superior positions, as well as giving orders, define the work situation of the lower positions and decide upon which individuals will be promoted up through the structure. In order to secure higher rewards and greater control over his job situation the individual must seek to satisfy his superiors. In other words, the people lowest on the scale and, therefore, in most contact with the clientele, have the greatest pressures to conform with the demands of their superiors. It is the wishes of the superiors, not the clientele, which govern the service giver's action.'
>
> (Hayes, 1979, p. 17)

Similarly, O'Hagan (1993) suggested that the traditional bureaucratic structure of many mental health services ensured users had little power to make decisions. Student nurses, according to Jones (1994, p. 6), occupied a position within hierarchies similar to that of service users: 'so far down the scale we don't register'.

In contrast, Mechanic (1968) noted the extent to which the lower ranking members of bureaucracies frustrated management proposals for change. Similarly, Sines (1994) regarded solidarity between nurses as a problem. Solidarity, however, is most usefully seen as a response to bureaucracies which ensure formal, rigid communications and offer little human support. Social experiments in which power was devolved to the front-line mental health workers, such as Towell and Harries' (1979) hospital innovation project, appear to be the products of a past age, when attempts, albeit flawed, were made to run organisations in a liberal democratic manner. Administrative rationality ensures little opportunity for the expression of human experience, which might challenge categorisation and control. Despite occasional protest, hierarchies generally ensure the skills of those at their base are either ignored or diminished. If psychiatric services were less hierarchical, it would be more difficult to maintain their central activities of coercion and control.

The position and role of those who are marginal to society has long been a topic of concern to psychoanalytical thinkers. The exclusion of someone who appears to think, feel and act differently from others may serve to preserve a sense of mass identity. Indeed, psychoanalytical theory suggests certain individuals are identified for this very reason. In so far as nurses seek actively to exclude people from their communities of origin, either on a long-term or short-term basis, they could be regarded as preserving mass identity and protecting those who are different.

Capitalism, coercion and control

The relationship between capitalism, coercion and control has been explored in several ways. Brown (1974) argued that mental sickness arises in a capitalist system in which people have to sell their own labour in order to survive; this results in the alienation of people from their own abilities, alienation of people from each other, and alienation from society. According to the Campaign Against Psychiatric Oppression (CAPO), alienated individualism, which arises from capitalist means and relations of production, lies at the root of much distress. The Socialist Patients Collective (SPC) (1993) argued that ill people have been exploited within capitalism, and that, once ill, they are further exploited by the pharmacological and insurance industries. In CAPO's and SPC's analysis, the coercion and control of individuals, under the guise of therapy, is an attempt to nullify the symptoms of capitalism and pacify class struggle.

In a similar vein, Navarro (1978) argues medicine serves to mystify the economic and political base of poor health, through positing individual problems and individual solutions rather than collective problems and collective solutions. In this sense, psychiatric medicine serves to maintain capitalism and associated relations of production. The illness-causing economic order of capitalism, termed 'iatrocapitalism' by SPC, can only be resolved through recognising illness as a form of protest against capitalism, and a potential weapon in the class struggle.

Scull (1989) and Sedgwick (1982), in contrast, acknowledged biological and psychological aspects of mental illness. Both saw psychiatric patients as unable to engage in waged labour. Scull (1989) argued that the closure of large psychiatric hospitals resulted from financial imperatives. Sedgwick (1982) was particularly critical of psychiatrists' social ambitions, and their attempts to dissociate themselves from the coercion and control of the poor, and to refocus on middle-class people with milder problems. (The same criticism could also be applied to community psychiatric nurses.) Scull and Sedgwick defend psychiatric institutions, and unlike CAPO and SPK do not criticise the contemporary conditions of labour. In an analysis of disablement, Oliver (1990) synthesises a number of positions. He acknowledges the biological dimension of illness, yet criticises institutions which house people who are excluded from the workforce, and recommends alliances between disabled people. In short, the centrality of coercion and control in psychiatric services is maintained by a complex of powerful forces, including rigid internal psychic order and equally rigid external economic order.

Power and mental health nursing education

This review has indicated ways in which the structure of the health service results from the sometimes conflicting, sometimes complementary, imperatives of the unconscious, formal administration and the healthcare market place. The primacy of social control in mental health services limits the extent to which 'formal interactive training' (Sines, 1994), for example counselling and other social skills, can be of any practical value. Given this situation, the author wishes, first, to indicate the importance of examining microsocial, mesosocial and macrosocial issues in some integrated way; secondly, to suggest the importance of examining a wide range of scientific, aesthetic and legal evidence within nurse education curricula; and thirdly, to discuss issues related to the ethics of listening, talking and acting in mental health nursing.

Microsocial

Empirical studies of nursing have often suggested the 'nurse–patient relationship' is a rarity, despite pronouncements concerning the proper task of nursing (Porter, 1992, 1993), or that the relationship, when it existed, was improper. A small number of studies have sought to understand interactions between nurses and users without making judgements about the kind of interactions that should exist. In Tilley's (1995) study of nurses' and users' views of mental health nursing, the importance of 'ordinary talk', about interests, hobbies, family and friends, as well as 'problem talk' was apparent. In a study of nursing from the perspective of both nurses and service users, Cormack (1983) suggested the centrality of basic humanity, such as simply being available, encouraging users to talk about their problems, being warm, understanding and sympathetic, encouraging confidence, security and optimism. In reality, the 'social skills' of nursing often amount to little more than simple humanity. The challenge to nurse education may be to preserve this humanity, rather than to teach nursing skills.

To this end, a number of strategies could be adopted. First, students' own experience could be seen as a resource. Students of mental health nursing could reflect upon their own experience of violence, coercion and control, both as perpetrator and victim; for example, occasions when they have felt discriminated against on the basis of gender, race, class, sexuality, or other life experience. Secondly, autobiographical accounts of psychiatric treatment, for example Millett's (1990) *The Looney Bin Trip*, could be regarded as forms of evidence, worthy of scrutiny in terms of aesthetic and theoretical merit. The 'art of accurate empathy' might be more effectively enhanced through an education focusing upon aesthetics, in particular fictional literature, storytelling, paintings and poetry, than one focusing on the reductionistic 'formal interactive training' (e.g. Sines, 1994).

Mesosocial

The relationship between sociology and psychiatry is presently often perceived in largely negative terms, but this obscures what has been a positive relationship and undermines the utility of sociology within psychiatry today. In particular, the sociology of institutions, communities, families and networks provides a useful basis for working with a wide range of organisations (Fleck, 1990; Eales, 1993; Eaton, 1994). As Clarke (1991) has suggested, it is useful to regard official inquiries as case studies. Novels by mental health nurses, in particular Sayers' (1988) *The Comforts of Madness* and Burrell's (1989) *Buster's Fired a Wobbler*, are full of telling insights into mental health nursing practice and education.

Macrosocial

Examination of the legal and policy-making processes related to mental health can be used to illustrate the relationship between parliament, pressure groups and public opinion. The issue of mental health is rarely far from legislative and policy fora, and examples of the process of legislative and policy change are therefore not difficult to find and follow. The relationship between nurses as agents of social control, and the manner in which nurses are supervised and regulated, deserves greater consideration. It is disconcerting that the cascade of change in health services appears to have limited opportunity for grassroots developments (Glenister, 1994).

Two macrosocial issues are worthy of brief note: democratisation and anti-oppressive practice. Democracy can be viewed as: (a) a principle of clinical practice; (b) a method of organising work in teams; and (c) a means of ensuring the accountability of local services to local people. However, the practice of this principle appears to have waned as post-war enthusiasm for popular administration has declined. Nevertheless, the pragmatic and moral imperatives concerning democratisation remain. The Mental Health Act Commission Fifth Biennial Report (HMSO, 1993) recommended a 'root and branch' approach to tackling racism in mental health services, and commended the Council for the Education and Teaching of Social Work's commitment to anti-discriminatory and antiracist practice. The Commission recommended educational programmes should at least promote awareness of racism in society, educate about antiracist practice, and convey theoretical knowledge about concepts of illness held by non-Western cultures.

Thus, an awareness of mental health and sickness in other cultures is a necessity, as is an awareness of racism's corrosive effect upon mental health within a predominantly white society. Given time and a willingness to explore multiple connections, the relationship between nurse and user, institution and community, and parliament, pressure groups and public opinion, might be illuminated, with educational and possibly therapeutic benefits. In short, macrosocial and political issues cannot simply be dismissed as context, since they are evident in mesosocial organisation and microsocial interaction.

The author advocates that students should develop critical appreciation of diverse forms of evidence which illuminate microsocial, mesosocial and macrosocial dimensions of mental health nursing practice. Following Habermas (1978), the author suggests that different forms of evidence could be examined according to different criteria. Aesthetic evidence could be contested with regard to its authenticity, technical evidence could be contested according to its truthfulness, and legal and moral judgements could be contested according to their rightfulness. This would correct the bias in favour of cognitive and psychomotor domains, and against the aesthetic domain, in mental health nursing education. To engage in this process would involve an ethical commitment to listening, speaking and acting. If dialogue between students and lecturers could be sufficiently developed, students might be able to take control of the curriculum, as formerly advocated by the statutory body for nurse education (English National Board, 1986). This dialogue might then be undertaken in more public places, such as meetings between staff and users, and the apparent necessity for cruder forms of coercion might diminish.

Conclusion

The assertion that care is the centre of nursing practice is challenged by a wealth of diverse evidence, including autobiography, official inquiries and reports. Unless mental health nurses face the reality of violence, coercion and control, attempts to empower users will be at best fatuous and at worst cynical. Given mental health nurses' and student mental health nurses' power to damage or enhance the quality of life of others, it is morally desirable that they should be aware of their capacity for control. Furthermore, the centrality of the process of gaining and maintaining control makes this a useful point on which to focus attempts to understand the organisation of mental health nurses and mental health services. If the shift towards 'evidence'-based healthcare involves discounting the experiental evidence of users, then it is simply a more sophisticated means for maintaining control of users and nurses. It is to be hoped that in the future, diverse forms of evidence, including both scientific and experiential evidence, will be contested through dialogue, and an open struggle for control will displace a simplistic and naive consensus concerning care.

References

Ackner, B. (1964) *Handbook for Psychiatric Nurses.* Ballière Tindall and Cassell, London.
Baruch, G. & Treacher, A. (1978) *Psychiatry Observed.* Routledge and Kegan Paul, London.
Barrett, P.M. (1992) Recovering humanity: towards an anti-psychiatric approach in nursing care. Unpublished RMN Project, Runwell Hospital, Wickford, Essex.
Barton, R. (1959) *Institutional Neurosis.* Wright, Bristol.
Barton, R. (1976) *Institutional Neurosis* 3rd edn. Wright, Bristol.
Beardshaw, V. (1981) *Conscientious Objectors at Work: Mental Nurses A Case Study.* Social Audit, London.
Benner, P. & Wrubel, J. (1989) *The Primacy of Caring: Stress and Coping in Health and Illness.* Addison Wesley, Menlo Park, California.
Blom-Cooper, L. (1992) *Committee of Inquiry into Complaints into Ashworth Hospital; Volumes I and II.* HMSO, London.
Bloor, D., McKeganey, N. & Flonkert, D. (1988) *One Foot in Eden: A Sociological Study of the Range of Therapeutic Practice.* Routledge, London.
Brown, P. (1974) *Towards a Marxist Psychology.* Harper and Row, New York.
Burrell, G. (1989) *Buster's Fired a Wobbler.* Penguin, Harmondsworth.
Campaign Against Psychiatric Oppression (Undated) *Introduction, Manifesto, and Demands.* CAPO, London.
Campbell, P. (1992) A survivor's guide to psychiatry. *Journal of Mental Health* 1, 117–122.
Chamberlin, J. (1988) *On Our Own: Patient Controlled Alternatives to the Mental Health System.* MIND, London.
Clarke, L. (1991) Ideological themes in mental nursing. In *Ethical Issues in Mental Health* (P.J. Barker & S. Baldwin eds). Chapman and Hall, London, pp. 27–44.
Clarke, L. (1994) Ethical psyche etc. in psych nursing. *Changes: International Journal of Psychology and Psychotherapy* 12 (2), 104–112.
Cormack, D. (1983) *Psychiatric Nursing Described.* Churchill Livingstone, Edinburgh.
Cullen, C. (1991) Ethics and clinical practice; a behavioural analysis. In *Ethical Issues in Mental Health* (P.J. Barker & S. Baldwin eds). Chapman and Hall, London, pp. 148–160.
Department of Health (1994) *Working in Partnership.* Department of Health, London.
Eales, M.J. (1993) Sociology and social psychiatry. In *Principles of Social Psychiatry* (D. Bhugra & J. Leff eds). Blackwell Science, Oxford.

Eaton, W.W. (1994) Social facts and the sociological imagination: the contribution of sociology to psychiatric epidemiology. *Acta Psychiatrica Scandinavica* **90** (Suppl. 385), 25–38.

English National Board (1986) *Syllabus of Training 1982: Professional Register – Part 3; Registered Mental Nurse*. HMSO, London.

Fleck, S. (1990) Social psychiatry – an overview. *Social Psychiatry and Psychiatric Epidemiology* **25**, 48–55.

Giddens, A. (1993) *Sociology*. Polity Press, Cambridge.

Glenister, D. (1994) Patient participation in psychiatric services. *Journal of Advanced Nursing* **19**, 802–811.

Habermas, J. (1978) *Knowledge and Human Interests*. Heinemann, London.

Harris, V. (1994) *Review of the Report of the Enquiry into the Care and Treatment of Christopher Clunis: A Black Perspective*. Race Equality Unit and National Institute of Social Work, London.

Hayes, E.W. (1979) Anti-psychiatric nursing. *Canadian Journal of Psychiatric Nursing* **20**, 16–18.

HMSO (1993) *The Mental Health Act Commission: Fifth Biennial Report 1991–1993*. HMSO, London.

HMSO (1995) *The Mental Health Act Commission: Sixth Biennial Report 1993–1995*. HMSO, London.

Horwitz, A.V. (1982) *The Social Control of Mental Illness*. Academic Press, New York.

Jones, H. (1994) All theory, no understanding. *Openmind* **69**, 6.

Jureidini, J. (1990) Projective identification in general psychiatry. *British Journal of Psychiatry* **157**, 656–660.

Lawrence, R. (1992a) Part 1: Torture and mental health: a review of the literature. *Issues in Mental Health Nursing* **13**, 301–310.

Lawrence, R. (1992b) Part 2: The treatment of torture survivors: a review of the literature. *Issues in Mental Health Nursing* **13**, 311–320.

Lovell, K. (1995) User satisfaction with in-patient mental health services. *Journal of Psychiatric and Mental Health Nursing* **2**, 143–150.

Lucksted, A. & Coursey, R.D. (1995) Consumer perceptions of pressure and force in psychiatric treatments. *Psychiatric Services* **46** (2), 146–152.

Main, S., Barron, McBride, I. & Austin, J.K. (1991) Patient and staff perceptions of a psychiatric ward environment. *Issues in Mental Health Nursing* **12**, 149–157.

Mechanic, D. (1968) *Medical Sociology: A Selected View*. Free Press, New York.

Millett, K. (1990) *The Looney Bin Trip*. Virago, London.

Navarro, V. (1978) *Class Struggle, The State and Medicine: An Historical and Contemporary Analysis of the Medical Sector in Great Britain*. Martin Roberson, London.

Nolan, P. (1993) *A History of Mental Health Nursing*. Chapman and Hall, London.

O'Hagan, M. (1993) *Stopover On My Way Home From Mars*. Survivors Speak Out, London.

Oliver, M. (1990) *The Politics of Disablement*. Macmillan, London.

Pembroke, L. (1991) Surviving psychiatry. *Nursing Times* **87** (49), 30–32.

Pollock, L. & West, E. (1984) On being a woman and a psychiatric nurse. *Senior Nurse* **1** (17), 10–13.

Porter, S. (1992) Institutional restraints upon education reforms: the case of mental health nursing. *Nurse Education Today* **12**, 452–457.

Porter, S. (1993) The determinants of psychiatric nursing practice: a comparison of sociological perspective. *Journal of Advanced Nursing* **18**, 1559–1566.

Sayers, P. (1988) *The Comforts of Madness*. Sceptre, London.

Scull, A. (1989) *Social Order/Mental Disorder*. Routledge, London.

Sedgwick, P. (1982) *Psycho politics*. Pluto Press, London.

Shepard, D. (1995) *Learning The Lessons: Mental Health Inquiry Reports Published in Britain Between 1969–1994*. Zito Trust, London.

Sines, D. (1994) The arrogance of power: a reflection on contemporary mental health nursing practice. *Journal of Advancd Nursing* **20**, 894–903.

Smith, G. (1986) Resistance to change in geriatric care. *International Journal of Nursing Studies* **23** (1), 61–70.

Socialist Patients Collective (1993) *Turn Illness into a Weapon*. Self-Publisher for Illness, Heidelberg.

Special Hospital Services Authority (1993) *Report of the Committee of Inquiry into the Death in Broadmoor Hospital of Orville Blackwood and a Review of the Death of Two Other Afro-Caribbean Patients*. SHSA, London.

Symonds, B. (1991) Sociological issues in the conceptualisation of mental illness. *Journal of Advanced Nursing* **16**, 1470–1477.

Tilley, S. (1995) *Negotiating Realities*. Avebury, Aldershot.

Towell, D. & Harries, C. (1979) *Innovation in Patient Care: An Action Research Study of Change in a Psychiatric Hospital*. Croom Helm, London.

United Kingdom Central Council for Nursing, Midwifery and Health Visiting (1996) *Guidelines for Professional Practice*. UKCC, London.

Wallcraft, J. & Read, J. (1992) *Guidelines for Empowering Users of Mental Health Services*. COHSE/MIND Publications, Banstead, Surrey.

5 Reflections from the Outside in: My Journey Into, Through and Beyond Psychiatric Nursing

Tessa Purkes

Introduction

This chapter will tell the story of my journey through mental health nursing, first as a student, then as a practitioner and now from the perspective of being outside. I shall attempt to address the question 'who is the mental health nurse?' by giving an account of my own version of the mental health nurse that was me, explaining the moves I made through this journey, my observations and concerns. This narrative will describe my personal response to nursing, to the 'profession', to the practice, and to the other nurses. I shall try to highlight the issues I found problematic in nursing practice by characterising the 'nurse' as I experienced her or him and relating this to how I made sense of 'nursing' in a more theoretical or conceptual sense.

In order to sustain the tensions I felt when I worked as a nurse I began to develop frameworks for thinking about what I was doing and what was going on around me. These frameworks, related to issues of power and responsibility, knowledge and language, then helped me to make sense of my journey through and then out of nursing by helping me to understand what I struggled with and why. This 'framing' became a way of coping with what ultimately I felt I could no longer remain part of.

Conceptualising the issues that I was faced with on a day-to-day basis helped me to make choices about where I was in my practice as a nurse, for example the choice to move out of a medical-biological framework of practice to a therapeutic community setting, and to move out of nursing altogether. Being able to frame the issues in nursing practice that were difficult for me helped me to distinguish between the personal and the political (organisational) dimensions of what I was doing. This process in turn enabled me to understand the part I played in different situations, and hence to construct different interpretations of those situations. This, I believe, helped me to be active rather than passive in trying to make sense of what I did and then through this to begin to act on new understandings rather than being bound by the old. As a result I could take greater responsibility for what I knew and what I then did.

The task of writing about my journey has been hard due to the difficulty I encountered in trying throughout the chapter to sustain the dual storylines of narrative (my moves in and out of nursing) and conceptual reflection (drawing on and exploring the frameworks that I found helpful in making sense of what I encountered as problematic).

Looking at the nurse and nursing practice: my perspective as a student

When I entered psychiatric nursing as a student I was completely unprepared for what I was to experience. My first experience on placement as a student nurse in a psychiatric ward was traumatic. I developed concerns about psychiatry, mental health nursing and hospitals that have stayed with me since; and the experience led me to make a commitment to work in the field of mental health. I realised after a few weeks that the assumptions I had made about the treatment, care and knowledge underpinning psychiatry's practice were unfounded. I was astonished at many aspects of the care of the people who were in hospital and the philosophy behind the treatments that were given. On one level it was the unmasked reality of human crisis, of abuse and suffering that I found traumatic; however, more difficult than this for me was the way in which this distress was interpreted and worked with.

One situation I remember was an occasion where having gone upstairs into a dormitory to do a job I interrupted a young man, Ben (a pseudonym), lying on his bed sobbing. Unsure as to whether he wanted me there or not I waited at the door. Without words he seemed to tell me that he did and I sat down beside him and held his hand while he continued to sob deeply, his anguish so powerful that I felt it would completely overwhelm him and perhaps me too. I said nothing. Neither did he. I stayed there as he became exhausted. After a while, a senior nurse came into the room looking for me. He looked quite taken aback by the obvious show of emotion and without hesitation asked me if Ben wanted any medication.

My feeling at the time was confusion since I could not at first understand the reaction of the nurse. I had been trying to communicate to Ben an acceptance of his sadness, an acceptance he had denied himself and been denied by others. Having spent some time with him and knowing him a little, I felt that he had become ashamed of his feelings, of himself and of his life and had stopped feeling able to show any emotion to others because of this. I knew I did not know what he was feeling or why, but what seemed to matter was that I did not judge him, and that I showed him my acceptance of him and what he was feeling. It seemed to me that Ben had only just found the courage to take off his mask, for himself and then for me when I walked in the door and entered in on his distress. I could not understand why his distress was seen to require tranquillising and suppressing. I felt that giving or offering medication encouraged Ben to put his mask back on again and would reaffirm his belief that he should not feel. In doing what I did I was using what I knew of Ben and my own personal theories of being human and in pain.

At the time I remember thinking that I had done something wrong, that I should have thought of medication too. Then as similar situations kept occurring I began to realise that I was probably using a different logic, had different ways of making sense of things. I began to wonder how I would survive as a nurse if I did make sense of what I was doing in ways quite different from those of other nurses. I realised, however, that my response to the personal experience of nursing would be unique to me, as that of others was to them, and that I would develop my own understandings to inform my practice.

One of my main frustrations as a student nurse was the difficulty I had relating the versions of the nurse in theory with the versions of the nurse in practice. Although the nurses I worked alongside often showed a sense of understanding what each person who required their help needed and an awareness of what had to be provided, I never found that this was reflected in the literature on nursing. Each nurse had their 'common sense' version of the nurse which bore little resemblance to the textbook versions espoused as containing yet another answer to the age-old problem of definition: 'What is the psychiatric nurse? What does she/he do? And why?'. The nurses I worked alongside were not following any identifiable models that explained their practice or interpretations. The exploration of the 'role' of the psychiatric nurse as far as I could see stayed in the class-rooms and textbooks, with practitioners wary of these questions, knowing that their practice could be neither well-defined nor explained in terms of theoretical principles and applications. Although some wards adopted nursing models such as the 'interpersonal relations' model or 'self-care' model, these had often been imposed on the ward team. They had not evolved as models close to the 'common sense' versions that nurses were working to.

Part of the problem, it seemed to me, lay in the position that nursing held in relation to other care-giving or therapeutic 'professions'. Nurses seemed to be struggling with the task of defining the purpose and meaning of what they were doing and hence were looking for answers by seeing themselves in relation to other professions. I felt that an uncritical reliance on know-ledge and theories borrowed from disciplines seen to be nursing's closest cousins, for example psychiatry, psychology and psychotherapy, was becoming apparent. As the role of the psychiatric nurse has changed over time, different knowledges have been seen as relevant to practice. The knowledge base which has imbued nursing practice has been, I believe, largely a combination of the ways other disciplines see their practice. Therefore, the understandings and ways of knowing that nursing now has have their roots in other disciplines and practices. For a number of reasons I felt that this was problematic.

I often wondered whether formal theory drawn from the more estab-lished disciplines was inadequate, since although it informed our prac-tice on a day-to-day level, through for example theories of symptom-management, behavioural techniques and counselling skills, it had little to say about the deeper concerns I encountered through being with people in crisis. The formal theories and ways of knowing that had been developed primarily through empirical science seemed to have few answers to the questions that arose from being with people in the often tragic, complex and insoluble situations of their lives. They gave me no understanding of, nor took any account of, what it is to be a person suffering in the world.

Psychiatry for example, has become aligned, largely, to what is known as the 'medical model' which promotes a systematic, rational and scientific approach to thinking about health and illness. It retains the deterministic perspective of cause and effect from which to make its diagnosis and hence treatment plans. Rather than moving away from the influence of the traditional scientific paradigm, psychiatry has chosen to stay, albeit in the shadows, within the safety of the dominant paradigm. It continues to embrace the dogma of scientism which assumes that only that which can be measured and tested can be given the status of reality. More questions are now being asked as to whether people can be understood in this way, with suggestions that a person must be placed in the context of his or her lived life (Dreyfus, 1987). On examination I concluded that a person's subjective experience was being excluded from view since it had no legitimate place as a source of knowledge.

I felt that the over-use of the scientific method in the understanding of human beings was doing more to hinder than to help me to make sense of mental distress. I felt it encouraged me to force the person into the moulds of the theories about them, fragmenting them into more accessible, less complex parts in order to enable 'understanding' of their abnormal functioning. This model of mental distress directed me to remove 'patients' from the complexity of their situation and to observe their behaviour in order to determine their psychopathology, while medicalising their distress by prescribing treatments and forcing them to surrender to medical expertise. I was, it seemed to me, to view myself as an expert practitioner, well-versed in the scientific and medical knowledge needed to get the mentally sick well or at least functional. I was to persuade the person to let go of their version of reality, of their thoughts and feelings, their stories, separating and disconnecting them from their understandings of themselves and their experience. To do this effectively I had to see myself as different, separate and apart from the person who was 'ill'. Like the scientist I was to be a distant, uninvolved observer.

Throughout my training I believed strongly that the complexity of working with people requires us to value diverse ways of knowing. Nursing practice as I saw it needed a variety of approaches to knowing, understanding and inquiry that were capable of reflecting the multiplicity of practice. Psychiatric nursing's dependence and reliance on the traditional scientific paradigm, through the disciplines of psychology, psychiatry and psychotherapy, was leading to an inadequate understanding of human being and human relationships. This obscured many of the other ways in which we 'know' and hence some of the rich, unquantifiable, subjective and personal facets of our practice. Instead of staying within the safe skirts of the scientific paradigm I felt that there was a need to develop other ways of knowing in order to remedy this imbalance.

For me nursing was about relationships, the interpersonal, the sense of partnership gained when working with people in ways that promoted and valued them as individuals with their own unique struggles. The role of the nurse as I saw it was to listen to the stories of people in pain and distress, to try to hear what had to be said, the story that had to be told. This, for me, was no different for people whose reality had shifted through attempting to live with their distress or inner transformation, people who had become immersed in their own reality with its own rules and patterns, values and meanings.

I saw my role as helping each person to try to make sense of their situation, themselves and their relationships in any way that they found helpful, meaningful and capable of giving them strength to start to untangle the knotted threads of their lives, to sustain themselves and the people around them. I tried to do this from the position of being me with my own subjectivity and perspectives holding a hand out to another; not an expert or learned professional. I tried working with people in ways that helped them to discover new meanings, realities and ways of re-authoring their lives. I tried to maintain a position of not-knowing from which I could reach out to people on their terms.

An example of how I did this was my work with a young man who was being nursed in a secure ward. When I first met 'Stephen' I was overwhelmed by his tragic story. I spent hours reading articles on psychological techniques, rehabilitation scales and institutional deprivation studies to try to find ideas for interventions that could possibly make a difference to his quality of life. I felt that there had to be some answers to the questions I was asking. I became aware, however, as I got to know Stephen and his situation that the interventions that I was learning about were not actually helping me to help him. They did not give me any answers. I realised that the situation was tragic in itself. Frustration took the place of my enthusiasm and energy and for a while I avoided spending time with him.

Primarily through talking to the other nurses on the ward and reflecting on my own concerns I began to understand that nursing was often about being alongside people in intolerable and unchangeable situations that sometimes could only be survived. This made me wonder how we as nurses should then be working with this reality to find hopeful and meaningful ways of working with people that could make positive differences to their lives. I realised then that the most powerful tool I had to use to do this was myself. Once I realised this I began to find new ways of working with Stephen which were about him and me and what I could offer which could be meaningful to him. One day we went to the sea since that was something he had always loved. I wanted to offer him some time out of his busy, lonely corridor for a while, some peace. I tried to promote what choice and control he had in little ways, tried to promote his sense of self. I wanted to help him to believe that he was still capable of feeling, of giving and receiving, of learning and teaching, of laughing and crying. This is what I thought I should be doing and what I called 'nursing' while I was with him.

I felt that the focus of nursing should be, not intervention, but rather being with people as they tried to pick up the pieces after whatever trauma they were in or had been through. The nurse's role was, I believed, to help people to make small changes and take small steps that embraced their own goals for themselves, rather than to 'manage' the illness or illness experience. Consequently nursing was more concerned with working with each person's subjective understandings of their distress or problem than with success or failure in terms of the ability to be 'cured' or 'rehabilitated'. Nurses could become too involved in 'doing for' rather than 'being with' people as they struggled to survive on a day-to-day basis; indeed the focus of the nurse's role as I saw it in practice was often more about ensuring compliance than about helping people to make real choices and decisions about their lives.

Becoming a practitioner: myself as nurse

After qualifying I became more and more aware of the disparity between how I wanted to be in my work and how I was able to be. The nurse, as I saw it, had a central and crucial role to play in the therapeutic alliance with the patient and his or her need for support, and yet had few tools available to do this work. The central interpersonal work so often had to be fitted in between other practical duties. This was a main reason why I decided to work in an environment which I thought would more closely fit with my own version of the mental health nurse – a therapeutic community. I thought of therapeutic communities as distinguishable from other hospital regimes, in respect of both the patients' greater degree of autonomy and involvement in their treatment and recovery, and an extended role for the nurse. I had many expectations of the therapeutic community environment as a mental health setting where I would be able to work with people in less constrained and more empowering ways.

When I had been in this new setting a while, however, I began to see that the former bastion of democracy was no longer that at all. All that was left was a shell of what had stood before, hollow and empty. I experienced there not a libertarian and supportive environment, but a combination of hierarchical, punitive and controlling structures. I tried hard to work positively within this environment, to integrate my version of the mental health nurse into the work of the ward. Unfortunately, the managers there saw my questions and exploration of practice as dissidence, and undermined, devalued and dismissed them.

Baron's (1987) analysis of a therapeutic community sheds light on some of the issues I faced. She details the potential for oppression in systems of care and therapy based on a libertarian rhetoric, the language of equality and participation often masking power dynamics. Baron draws particular attention to the central place of leadership, especially charismatic leadership in these forms of community, and to the danger of abuses of power that can arise if the leader has contradictory or manipulative goals.

I struggled to work with the differences between my way of trying to practise and the dynamics of this setting, but eventually could no longer do so without losing my individuality and self-respect. I felt I had no choice but to leave. Despite having chosen an environment I thought would be conducive to my ideas about nursing, I found that as a psychiatric nurse I would not be permitted the freedom I desired to work with people in the way that I wanted to. I was tired of trying to explain myself and tired of trying to fit in to places I had no affinity with, held together by structures I could not believe in.

I had learned from my teachers that there are many different versions of the psychiatric or mental health 'nurse'. My version, I came to believe, was at odds with the main established versions no matter where I worked. I was called 'naive', 'idealistic', 'out of touch'. Working in environments soaked in values that I did not share, and did not wish to share, forced me to face what it was that I did want in my work as 'nurse'. I discovered fairly early on that the nurse was not a free agent, could never be in current circumstances. The constraints of the bureaucratic institution, of nursing's subservient relationship to medicine, of the limiting and dubious knowledge base of psychiatry and psychiatric nursing, of our own uncertainty about ourselves and our skills, of lack of respect from other professions and lack of personal and professional authority to create meaningful change: all these obstructed our freedom to be what we wanted to be.

My role frequently got lost within the agendas of value-laden assessment procedures, medical treatment, restraint and containment of emotional chaos. People's struggles were often decontextualised from their lives, social circumstances, family and culture. The process of medicalising distress cut people off from finding their own patterns, seeking out their own meanings and finding their own solutions. Psychiatric professionals often intervened in ways that prevented those who came for help from using their own resources. They did so by mobilising powerful professional strengths, for example medication, invasive treatments, therapies, observation and control, while simultaneously demobilising the patients' own strengths. Psychiatrists and nurses seemed largely to devalue the process of people being involved in and indeed responsible for their own mental health and well-being.

While I was working as a nurse I struggled against the use of labels for people's distress, but found it impossible to work without them completely because I was working within the medical paradigm. I was also concerned about the language that nurses used with regard to the people they were supposed to be helping, and the connections between knowledge and power. Through reading about discourse analysis and language I had come to understand that language not only describes our realities, it also constitutes them, shaping our social relationships and identities (Fairclough, 1992). Language indicates what counts as knowledge, placing people within texts as subjects and objects, as 'knowers' and 'known', establishing relationships between them.

Susko's (1994) work on problems inherent in the language of psychiatry helped me make sense of my unease. He contrasts the use of the 'caseness' approach with the 'narrative' approach when working with people who are labelled psychiatrically. The 'caseness' approach means the process of objectifying a person in the medical system, i.e. the person becoming a case or being perceived as one. This approach consists of identifying target symptoms, making a diagnosis and intervening to stop or manage symptoms. It labels the 'madness' experience as a disease entity by identifying negatively valued symptoms. The 'narrative' approach is an alternative to the caseness approach which allows people to find their own meanings and create their own explanations from their 'madness' experience.

Implicit in the 'caseness' approach is a power disparity reflecting the separation of 'knower' and 'known'. This disparity does not occur in the narrative approach. There, symbols, imagery and metaphor can be used to try to explain the madness or distress experience, and make it accessible to another to share. A transformative, integrative or restorative effect can occur through using the narrative approach. Susko believes that this approach can provide an alternative frame of reference for attempting to understand the 'madness' experience and can allow a person to establish the discourse from which a dialogue can develop.

I found awareness of discourse particularly relevant to the exploration of power and responsibility in nursing and psychiatry. Foucault (1975, 1977) wrote of the close relationship between knowledge and power, highlighting the development of discourses that attempted to define certain forms of reason and knowledge as having a greater truth status than others. Science and medicine were two of these 'objective' reality discourses accorded a higher status than other 'local', 'popular' or 'indigenous' knowledges. These ideas when applied to the science of psychiatry go some way towards explaining why the objective discourses of case studies, assessments, diagnostic labelling and problem-solving are so predominant and why the personal, relational and temporal aspects of the experience of being in crisis have been lost.

Susko's (1994) work again is useful in drawing connections between these opposing discourses, with respect to the practice of working with people in distress. He believes that in the diagnostic process of labelling a transfer of ownership takes place:

'With naming comes a transfer of *ownership* of the person's mind and body to the professional. If someone's brain is diseased, that individual ceases to be viewed as a responsible owner of his or her mind/body.'

(Susko, 1994, p. 93)

Here responsibility, not only for the illness and problem but also for the lived life, is seized by the one who names. In this process, according to Susko (1994, p. 93):

'Nurses and attendants, as the representatives of the medical system function as the new owners of the patient's body/mind ...'

In the narrative approach, the person keeps the power of definition and explanation, thereby holding onto responsibility for naming and making sense, retaining ownership and not relinquishing control to the 'experts'. The work I have outlined here helped me to position nurses as keepers of the language and values of the medical system within the person's/ patient's world and daily reality, helping me to understand something I had noted in practice: the sense of ownership expressed by nurses regarding 'their patients'.

Moving on and out of nursing: where I moved to

I now work as a team leader with a voluntary not-for-profit organisation. This organisation provides services, in particular supported accommodation, for people who have long-standing mental health problems. I was attracted to the voluntary sector because it seemed to allow much of what I had struggled to do in nursing: to personalise the relationships, to de-stigmatise, to support and challenge (and to be supported and challenged) in ways that encouraged growth and change.

My organisation aims to provide normal living facilities in ordinary houses in the community, for people who cannot independently sustain a tenancy. It also aims to help people to become part of their communities again through the use of ordinary and valued activities and amenities. It places emphasis on respecting the needs, ambitions, preferences and choices of each person who receives support. The support for tenants comes from support workers whose primary task is to enable tenants to experience ordinary life. This can involve helping to reduce isolation, promoting the exercise of rights, improving self-esteem and self-identity, helping with ordinary domestic living, encouraging respect for each other, and developing skills both in and outside the house.

The philosophy guiding the work I do parallels approaches such as normalisation and social role valorisation in advocating the right of everyone to an ordinary life. It entails respect for the rights to self-determination, to decide for oneself, to make mistakes, to be independent, dependent, and/or interdependent, and 'the dignity of risk'. This approach recognises the need to help people to be aware of the disadvantages and risks embedded in their choices (Ramon, 1991). In my work now I try to help people to discard the devalued images of themselves and to reverse the process of institutionalisation and labelling, by positively valuing their individuality. I feel that I am now able to work in ways that return to people a sense that they are in control of their lives. I am often challenged by the need to work with chaos, uncertainty and doubt, stemming from the often chaotic nature of life itself and from living in a world that presents so many challenges to our desire for order, regulation and structure.

In my work now I feel that I am free to find supportive rather than coercive ways of working with people. I use myself and my own know-ledge of each person rather than 'expert' or 'professional' knowledge of disorder or disease. I can attend to the person and how they make sense of their world, their emotional and practical lives and their reality or realities. Therein lies the challenge.

Dr Edward Podvoll's (1990) *The Seduction of Madness – A Revolutionary Approach to Recovery at Home* captures a sense of the kind of work I am trying to do:

> 'Empowered in this way to take mental health into our own hands, we need no longer rely simply on 'experts' to banish madness. By understanding the importance of environment, an ordinary home can become a natural place for healing.'
>
> (Podvoll, 1990, p. 318)

Podvoll challenges the assumed necessity of the 'industrialisation of mental health', and describes a new approach to care and support for people with mental health problems. The book rises above the predictable pessimism of traditional views on helping people with long-standing mental health problems by focusing on the individual's potential for 'islands of clarity' and even recovery. The chapters on basic attendance, discovering islands of clarity, and creating a therapeutic home provide arguments for the therapeutic potential of ordinary homes and ordinary people as the means and basis for the support of those experiencing 'madness'.

Podvoll (1990) describes the home as an ideal place for 'recovery', and the role of the 'attendant' as opposed to the 'professional' or 'expert'. The skills of basic attendance are described as abilities: to listen; to go at another's pace; to be responsive and empathic; to be practically and emo-tionally able; to be able to relate to the wider environment of the person, i.e. the house, family, friends; to be able to work as part of a team yet bring and have confidence in one's individual abilities and qualities; to be interested and interesting; to see the person one is working with as an individual; to be able to focus on the individual rather than any disorder, disease or label; to have patience and tolerance; and to see work as both giving and receiving.

The Seduction of Madness details the complexities of the work that can be done and is being done to promote positive mental health with people who have long-standing mental health problems, and to enhance their quality of life. It proposes the values of human intimacy and relatedness, respect, compassion and openness as foundations for recovery, self-control and self-mastery. In my view this model of basic attendance provides a tenable vision of care and support for people who experience severe mental or emotional distress, as a radical option for the development of nursing. Within this model, nurses would play a role more like that of the support worker, being alongside the person, 'working with' rather than 'doing to'. 'Basic attendance' is not simply 'supporting' another person; it also involves turning over to them the means by which they can support themselves. The emphasis would be on practical help and emotional support. Is it possible that the new 'nurse' of the future will play the role of 'attendant' within this enlightened framework of support rather than control?

How I see nursing practice and nurses now: from the outside looking in

My version of the nurse feels most at home doing what I do now. In the light of the current debate on the provision of services for people with mental health needs, and the growing confusion about the nurse's role, I believe that the work being done by some of the voluntary organisations offers a great challenge to the nursing profession. Partnership rather than paternalism is now recognised as being more appropriate in most spheres of health promotion and practice.

Today the large psychiatric institutions are closing down and the world of nursing as it was is dying. Change, uncertainty and confusion are now hallmarks of a world that was so certain and predictable. Mental health policy changes have hit psychiatric nursing hard, and the profession is now struggling to make a niche for itself in the community and in what is left of the institutional services. The future is insecure, the past devalued and destroyed. The identity of the psychiatric nurse is being called into question as the role of the hospital in today's contract climate is challenged. The profession has to look carefully at its remit and at the skills its practitioners use and will need in the future.

One track being followed by some nurses is the pursuit of professionalism through more specialised treatments and techniques such as behavioural therapy, nursing diagnoses and various psychotherapeutic interventions. This aim to develop a professional, expert and esoteric body of knowledge to be kept from, yet applied to, the 'patient' is antithetical to the ideals of partnership and reciprocity identified as the way forward in health care (World Health Organisation, 1978). Indeed, the pursuit of professionalisation might create more barriers between nurses and patients or users, rather than breaking them down. Olshansky (cited in Brandon, 1991) argues that this could well be the case. Olshansky writes, on the subject of normalisation work and professionals:

'First, professionals, by training, are committed to treating pathology and abnormality. One might say they always see pathology and abnormality even where none exists ... Second, professionals too often develop a sense of superiority to the people they help. Enjoying feelings of superiority, they somehow lose interest and faith in the capacity of their 'inferiors' to change, to grow. Moreover, they expect less from inferior persons ... Third, professionals tend to see only the 'inner space', the intrapsychic. The only experiences they value are the clinical ones, where they are in control and their contacts are brief. The experiences outside the clinic seem to them of little value ... Fourth, professionals are imprisoned by habits. They prefer to do what they have done. It is easier and more comfortable to treat pathology as they have been doing and as they have been trained to do. The principle of normalisation is a challenge to change their focus and habits.'

(Brandon, 1991, p. 41)

This passage reflects fairly accurately how I see the work of the majority of health professionals, now that I am outside the 'profession'.

Another challenge to nursing comes from research on users' views of psychiatric services. According to Rogers *et al.* (1993) the model of practice preferred by users stresses personal contact and understanding and rejects specialised treatments and techniques. Their study describes the high value clients place on the informality and the flexibility of the voluntary sector. These aspects valued by users conflict with trends within professional training which focus on creating increasingly 'specialised' services and modes of intervention. Rogers *et al.* (1993) propose that

'High levels of 'skill' and 'expertise' whether in psychological therapies, medicine or nursing, run counter to the emphasis on *deskilling* which is implied by what users identify as being beneficial: that is, if professionals were to approximate to the conception preferred by users, they would have to shed most or all of their pretentions towards specialised knowledge.'

Mental health services also face pressures to acknowledge individuals' rights to define their own needs, and to see the recipients of services as equal partners. Psychiatric nursing, to my mind, should be looking for ways to involve users in determining what they need from nursing, and ways to shift the current imbalance of power. I believe that the legitimacy of medical interventionism in the field of mental health likewise is increasingly being challenged.

With the development of community care, different agencies have to work together to plan service provision to meet the identified needs of clients and service users. Nurses now have to negotiate their role and responsibilities with other professionals in a way they never had to before. Although community care is about shifting the environment of care from institutions to the community, it is also about changing the way health and social care/support needs are met. For this to work, and for true partnership to be achieved, professionals have to take a quite different view of their roles. Professionals now need to see themselves as working 'with' people to meet their health or social needs, rather than 'for' them. Brandon (1991) argues that the principles of normalisation, not the medical model style of 'helping', should now direct professional work.

My experience is that these developments are not happening in institutions. Nurses seem to be refusing to give up their old ways of thinking and working with people even when working in the community. Like Olshansky's professionals, they 'prefer to do what they have done.' Not only are nurses not embracing a new philosophy of practice for their work in the community, I fear that they are becoming the agents of the new strategies for control and surveillance in the community. Bean and Mounser (1993) assert that the community is seen increasingly as an extension of the mental hospital, with the new supervision registers and community treatment orders/care orders marking a strengthening of psychiatry's structural position within the community.

Although these developments stem largely from reactive government policies, fuelled by the power of the media, mental illness professionals have also played their part in sustaining old myths about the mentally ill and clamping down on innovative thinking in the field of mental health provision. There seems to be an investment in keeping alive old power relations, old dependencies and old relationships. I see a future in which nurses in the community act as knights roaming the land to keep the old versions alive, the old established order intact, even though their castles have crumbled.

The 'contract culture' that now pervades our organisation's work with the statutory services has produced a shift in relationships. The contract has become a new means of continuing the old versions of patients and care in new forms. When people are discharged from hospital their past histories still drag behind them in the form of old records, labels and professional judgements. I believe that the work done by the voluntary agencies is being infiltrated by the old discourses of power and knowledge through required use of assessments, labels and programmes of care as part of purchasing agreements. These agreements increasingly prescribe what should be done and the way it should be done. The new discourses being developed through work with user groups on human rights, normalisation and integration, are still vulnerable when set up against the old medical and social control discourses. They are frequently dismissed as unprofessional or nonsensical.

I think that future systems should seek to transcend old boundaries and barriers, not reinforce them. My view, reinforced by the proposals made by Rogers *et al.* (1993), is that mental health services should be developing new systems based on partnership, ordinary equal relationships, empowerment, mutual aid and self-help, advocacy and self-advocacy, with a commitment to the de-marginalisation of those who use mental health services. A post-medical user-led service which could be a radical alternative to the present psychiatric services may only come about through reduction of the power of current mental illness professions.

Implications for education

Having described my journey in and out of psychiatric nursing and offered thoughts on certain areas that I found to be problematic within the practice and theory of psychiatric nursing – areas that, even now that I have left nursing, still impinge on my work and the people I work with – I want to relate these thoughts to changes which would have to be made if nursing education is to respond to some of the above challenges.

Most importantly, I believe that each person's experience of nursing is unique. We need an individualised education system that recognises this and helps each nurse to develop as a 'reflective practitioner' (Schön, 1983). This education system should develop the use of reflective thinking for exploration of personal values and meanings inherent in our work. It should focus on the relational, personal and subjective ways of knowing so that nurses can begin early on to recognise themselves in the nursing experience. Journal-keeping with opportunities to reflect on the personal material thus generated can go some way towards encouraging the student nurse to do this. Critical thinking should be promoted to challenge current regimes of practice and ways of thinking about practice, to allow room for development and change. Students should be taught less about how things are, perpetuating worn out ways; more about how they may be, could be or should be.

Each institution and working environment has its own values and philosophy which influence the development of its members by ordering actions and expectations. It is crucial for the new nurse to find a place that suits her and her beliefs if she is to avoid being negatively overwhelmed. The new nurse should be enabled to test out the contexts and values in different environments, to see if she can work within them. Nurse education should therefore help the student to manage the tensions between personal and organisational forces in the workplace, helping her to realise the impact of organisational barriers. This can involve allowing students to develop frameworks for thinking about what they as nurses do. Discourse analysis and theories of deconstruction can serve as tools for this exploration, helping students to recognise power and knowledge mediated by language and their effects on nurses and the people they are trying to help. Without some such understanding new nurses are more vulnerable to organisational forces which might render them passive objects rather than active players.

I believe that an education system should promote an awareness of the problematic nature of helping in psychiatric contexts so that students are aware of how psychiatric institutions coerce both them and the patients/ users. Nurses need to be aware of coercive practices, including use of rhetoric and verbal persuasion. The educational institutions need to be attentive to the power relationships of the new political and therapeutic climate in which psychiatric nursing is now immersed, given moves into alternative environments of care with new models and theories of treatment and support, and different power relationships and strategies of control. They must have an investment in the relocation of power away from the professionals and towards the service users; in other words, an investment in transcending traditional elitism. Nurses should not be taught that they know best; instead they should be provided with opportunities to explore and share their own vulnerabilities in order to be able to take on working with anyone else's. If these challenges are met it may be possible that psychiatric nursing can become part of the future in mental health services rather than being an anchor to the past.

References

Baron, C. (1987) *Asylum to Anarchy*. Free Association Books, London.
Bean, P. & Mounser, P. (1993) *Discharged from Mental Hospitals*. Macmillan Press, London.

Brandon, D. (1991) The implications of normalisation work for professional skills. In *Beyond Community Care. Normalisation and Integration work* (S. Ramon, ed.). Macmillan Press, London, pp. 35–56.

Dreyfus, H. (1987) Foucault's critique of psychiatric medicine. *The Journal of Medicine and Philosophy* **12**, 311–333.

Fairclough, N. (1992) *Discourse and Social Change*. Polity Press, Cambridge.

Foucault, M. (1975) *The Archaeology of Knowledge*. Tavistock, London.

Foucault, M. (1977) *Discipline and Punish*. Allen Lane, London.

Podvoll, E.M. (1990) *The Seduction of Madness. A Revolutionary Approach to Recovery at Home*. Harper Collins, New York.

Ramon, S. (1991) *Beyond Community care. Normalisation and Integration Work*. Macmillan Press, London.

Rogers, A., Pilgrim, D. & Lacey, R. (1993) *Experiencing Psychiatry. User Views of Services*. Macmillan Press, MIND, Basingstoke.

Schön, D. (1983) *The Reflective Practitioner*. Temple Smith, London.

Susko, M.A. (1994) Caseness and narrative: contrasting approaches to people who are psychiatrically labelled. Challenging the Therapeutic State Part Two: Further Disquisitions on the Mental Health System. *Journal of Mind and Behavior* **15**, 87–112.

World Health Organisation (1978) *Alma Alta International Conference on Primary Health Care*. WHO, Geneva.

6 Reflections of a Senior Nurse Manager

Linda C. Pollock

Introduction

When asked to contribute my perceptions of psychiatric nursing to this book I accepted the invitation willingly. The opportunity to distil my views seemed a welcome diversion from my 'normal' routine. The approach I have taken has been to reflect retrospectively on my career. In standing back to look at my different roles within psychiatric nursing, I have tried to document what I learned from my various work experiences, and to highlight the key influences that have shaped me into the psychiatric nurse that I am today. As with all retrospection, wisdom has perhaps been superimposed on my reflections – I leave you, however, to be the judge of that!

I am a Nursing Director on a Board within a Trust, and am a General Manager. The fact that I was once a 'real' nurse surprises some, and I am often asked 'as an administrator, do you not miss "hands-on" nursing work?' In truth, many of my decisions directly affect nursing staff and patients, I feel therefore that I still have a major influence on what goes on at the bedside. I must admit too, that I get angry at being described as an 'administrator' – the term implies paper shuffling and blindly carrying out instructions from above. I do not indulge in either of the latter two activities, and my day-to-day work involves dealing with people, reviewing and assessing situations and priorities, and thoughtful decision making. All of these skills I began learning in my 'basic' nurse training days.

Looking back to the start

I left school in 1971 to take up my first hospital job, as a nursing auxiliary in a surgical ward. I was thrown in the deep end, with no induction or orientation, left to draw on my girl guide experiences and common sense. In my first week, I saw someone die and gave first aid to someone having an epileptic fit in the bathroom. I was planning to go to university and study geography, but I enjoyed the nursing work, particularly dealing with people, so much that I went to see the matron to arrange to begin training as a nurse, instead of going to university.

The matron told me about the 'integrated' degree course that ran at

73

Edinburgh University. It was a combined nurse training with a BSc degree, over a 4½-year period. Very few nurses entered nursing via these degree courses, so this route into nursing was unusual and unconventional. The training was lengthy (compared with the 3 years undertaken by traditional nurses), but I was excited by the idea of being a student and sampling university life as well as doing nursing.

I didn't think about doing psychiatric nursing at that stage at all. Funny, isn't it, my career into nursing via an academic pathway was triggered by accident and the good advice of the matron at the infirmary. To her I owe a debt of gratitude. I don't regret having done 'general' nursing first – it gives you a good grounding and allows you to have confidence in dealing with patients' physical needs and medical emergencies, many of which can arise in the psychiatric setting.

It was a wonderful experience being a student and studying a range of topics and subjects not related to nursing. The experience was literally mind expanding, and it was a great opportunity to be a student in the 1970s – getting involved in demonstrations and marches, not to mention parties and late night heavy debates about feminism and socialism! If you're prepared to wait longer to become a staff nurse, I'd recommend doing a 'degree' course – there are now a lot to choose from.

Striving for the ideal

What a preparation that degree course turned out to be: almost 5 years of academic study with mentors and tutors who were, and who remain, some of the most stimulating and thought-provoking figures in nursing. The training I received was similar to that envisaged for Project 2000 students (Hallet *et al.*, 1995), based in a higher educational setting, with an emphasis on health and community care; further, it was designed to produce reflective and articulate practitioners. At the time, traditionally-trained nurses believed that the course was intended to produce managers and high flyers who did not really want to nurse. The research evidence has shown otherwise (Sinclair, 1987), confirming that most degree nurses willingly stay in practical work, most often in the community setting. Such evidence will be comforting to supporters of Project 2000 (White, 1995; Bentley, 1996), who wish to see more community nurses, and a reduced wastage and improved retention rate for nursing. It seems that degree courses are good at teaching new nurses about 'the ideal' care to be given. I believe that the way these ideals are presented, by individuals with passion and enthusiasm, yet also with a sense of what can be achieved in reality, is crucial to the student nurse.

I believe that the degree course produced thoughtful and caring practitioners with a value base firmly focused on patient care. I was provided with a theoretical knowledge base which has held me in good stead and prepared me well for a nursing career. I was always taught that the patient comes first, that dignity and respect for individuals is crucial and that high quality care is the key to the service that we deliver. We had a course for a whole term, 10 weeks, on 'the role of the patient'. I have never forgotten the messages we learned in those early days, and I firmly believe that all foundation courses should emphasise these tenets.

Questioning the status quo

I was encouraged to question and challenge existing practices and more importantly, to find solutions to problems. The grounding I received was as much due to the lecturers who inspired me as to the formal curriculum and course assignments. Lecturers who taught and influenced me included Annie Altschul, Rosemary Crow, Lisbeth Hockey, Edith Notman, Ruth Schrock, Margaret Scott Wright, Billy Thompson and Alison Tierney. Closer scrutiny of the names shows that some of our best psychiatric nurses and eminent researchers influenced me in those formative years as a novice nurse. In choosing your degree course then, I would recommend that you consider the lecturers, their interests and their publication track records. They will strongly influence what is put into, and thus what you will get out of, the nursing degree course that you choose.

It's difficult to know if my inquisitive attitude was stimulated by my time at university (because the nature of doing a degree course was that it did encourage me to explore and search for answers), or if my aptitude for challenging and examining issues is a trait which is naturally mine. What I do know, is that it is important that all nurses acquire the ability to review and scrutinise the wealth of data that is presented. Nurses need to distil information and then present it in an understandable and logical format, in care plans or reports, and I learned these skills well on the degree course. Writing and recording can be seen as an unnecessary chore by so many traditionally-trained nurses.

I've found too that, compared with colleagues who have completed traditional nursing courses, I am more comfortable and confident in asserting my point of view, more able to speak up for patients, and to argue with colleagues (who have had university-level education). Traditionally-trained nurses do have these skills of course. I only wish that all nurses were equipped with such professional convictions, and that from the beginning of their training, they could be encouraged to ask senior managers or practitioners to justify their opinions and explain the reasons for actions. Nurses would be less passive and nursing generally would feel more in control of its destiny. Basic training for nursing should encourage questioning and teach nurses to be assertive and professional in their arguments.

Theory into practice

My early experience of psychiatric nursing practice was in a therapeutic community setting in 1972. There had been much publicity about various atrocities in psychiatric hospitals (Martin, 1984), and I approached this practice placement with some trepidation. However, the psychiatric hospital was one that had been developed and shaped by Maxwell Jones (Manning, 1989), a pioneer of the therapeutic community movement, and it was an exciting and innovative place to learn. Patients ate with staff in a joint dining room and staff behaviour was questioned by patients at 'sensitivity' and 'patient council' meetings. Such forums encouraged nurses to justify their actions and forced us truly to listen to and take account of patients' views. Again the university tutors, Annie Altschul and Ruth Schröck, were important influences. They encouraged us continuously to put the theory of patient care into practice, and supported us to articulate our experiences and make sense of what we were doing. The Dingleton experience stimulated my interest in psychiatric nursing, and made me realise that putting patients' emotional and social needs at the centre of nursing interactions was the secret of 'good' nursing care.

Setting standards

My next experience of psychiatry was in a traditional psychiatric hospital. As in the first hospital, the placement was in a long-term ward, but here 'institutionalisation' (Goffman, 1975), of both staff and patients, was evident. All patients received white, sugared tea out of a large teapot. The ward routine consisted of tasks, queuing for medication, meals, baths, allocation of communal clothing, and the patients were destined to live passive, boring lives in front of a TV and radio (both were constantly on).

I have no doubt that the differences in the organisation and therapeutic *milieu* of the two wards were related to the views and standards set by the respective charge nurses. Research done since my early experiences has shown that the charge nurse is key in relation to setting standards and maintaining a high quality of environment for patients (Buchan *et al.*, 1993). My differing psychiatric experiences proved that to me.

I therefore applaud the UKCC's emphasis on career-long development and requirement that nurses demonstrate that their knowledge is up-to-date before they re-register. This, along with the encouragement of managers to set annual objectives for their staff, undertake appraisals, and put in place supervisory systems, should prevent nurses from becoming 'burned out', performing poorly and creating untherapeutic settings. My personal experience is that individual benefits and satisfaction, as well as patient gain, are to be had from acquiring new knowledge and skills.

The next step: the attraction of emotional distress

By 1976, I had finished my integrated degree course and had gained my BSc, RGN and Certificate of District Nursing. I loved the course and enjoyed most of my placements. Throughout my general nurse (RGN) training however, I was appalled at two things. The first was the massive insults that bodies are subjected to by mutilating surgery and aggressive therapeutic interventions. The physical care given could not be faulted, but the attention paid to the psychological effects of treatments, and indeed to helping relatives cope with the sequelae of treatments, was minimal.

Secondly, talking to patients and carers, even the recently bereaved, was not well done. In some areas talking to patients was actively discouraged (I was often told to go and clean cupboards during quiet spells rather than develop rapport with patients); in other wards, difficult patients were avoided or labelled (Menzies, 1960). I distinctly remember, in the first ward that I staffed, being told by the junior doctor to go and 'deal with' the relatives: he'd just informed them that their mother had died – suddenly, unexpectedly, traumatically, after an overdose. I was left to mop up the pieces, and I did so inadequately. I did not have the ability to deal with the emotional distress of my patients and/or carers.

My first staff nurse job was in the poisons unit, a specialist area of a very large general hospital. The wards, one male and one female, dealt exclusively with patients who had been poisoned (accidental poisonings as well as attempted suicides), who were admitted directly to us from accident and emergency. This field was not an attractive or desirable specialism in which to work but I found it exciting and it provided varied opportunities to develop technical nursing skills. Some patients needed intensive nursing care, e.g. the unconscious patient who had overdosed with barbiturates and was on a ventilator; other patients had taken overdoses of amytryptilene and were on ECG machines. We were trained to 'extend' our role and take bloods. Some of the patients were depressed, usually those who had taken the anti-depressants. Often they had been prescribed the drugs and overdosed when, after days without any improvements and feeling they were 'untreatable', they tried to end it all.

Some of the accidental poisonings were firemen (poisoned by fumes from burning furniture), or family members who had by accident drunk poisons (e.g. bleach or paraquat). Most of the 'accidental' poisonings were drug addicts who had overdosed on morphine or a mixture of substances. The wards had a constant stream of 'regulars', who intermittently took overdoses, often after drinking alcohol and usually after arguments with partners. The chances were that these overdosers would eventually kill themselves. This pattern of behaviour became known as 'para-suicide' (Kreitman, *et al.*, 1969) and the individuals fascinated me. I couldn't understand why they kept trying to kill themselves.

All patients were seen by a psychiatrist before discharge from the wards, yet although the ward received over 200 admissions per month, few were transferred to psychiatric care. I was amazed that the majority of admissions were considered mentally normal. Surely such behaviour was a sign of emotional distress and need for help? Yet so few of those individuals were referred on or offered any follow-up. I was also intrigued because it wasn't necessarily the most serious overdose cases who were referred to psychiatry. It seemed common sense that on-going support to the 'para-suicides' would have been worth trying, to help reduce the repeat rate. I was sure that these people, who seemed to be crying out for help, could indeed be helped: yet no ongoing support was offered to 'the regulars'. I decided at this point to go and do my psychiatric nurse training – I felt that

I would gain a better understanding of mental illness and human behaviour and learn how to counsel. I intended to return to general nursing, armed with such skills and knowledge, and to use those skills to give better psychological support to patients and families.

Comfort and confidence with psychological disturbance

I did my psychiatric nurse training in Edinburgh. It did help me understand the mind and gave me confidence to deal with people whose thinking was disturbed and who behaved abnormally. Psychiatric nurse training, on the whole, was a disappointment. I didn't have the same academic stimulation as I had at university, In retrospect, it must have been difficult for tutors to match up to the Annie Altschuls and Ruth Schröcks of this world! Also, I think I had difficulty in adjusting from the high tech, life saving pace of the suicide ward to sitting and talking to people in emotional distress. I thought many of the experienced psychiatric nurses with whom I worked were lazy or uninterested. In years to come, I came to understand that some of these staff were unmotivated because they were 'burned out' and had given up trying to change the system (Lemmer & Smits, 1989). I vowed that, whatever my role, I would try to support and motivate colleagues, not oppress and repress them.

On reflection, my psychiatric training period was not all bad. The good wards had good charge nurses, who were good role models, and I worked with colleagues and peers (from clinical psychology, social work, occupational therapy and medicine, as well as nursing) who were interested and motivated, and from whom I learned a great deal. I learned to understand negative experiences and the importance of retaining an optimism and consistency of approach to help individuals through their distress. Two influences sustained my interest in psychiatry. One was the patients themselves – I could see that I was able to help some patients develop and change for the better. I seemed to be drawn to working with patients 'labelled' as 'long term', who had been rejected by others and were some of the most distressed and demanding of patients. They were like a magnet to me, and I found the challenge of developing relationships with them fascinating and rewarding. I'll never forget some of those patients.

Group psychotherapy and clinical supervision

The second influence was the therapeutic *milieu* in which I worked. I trained at a time when group therapy was in vogue and I was incredibly lucky to gain experience in group and individual psychotherapy. I developed this interest in groupwork and, in the evenings, did an intensive 2-year course, in small group psychotherapy, at the Institute of Human Relations. This training in the dynamics of psychotherapy has provided me with skills and confidence in listening, managing and dealing positively with people in group situations; I still use these skills.

Training as a therapist also highlighted for me that all nurses need to have clinical supervision while they practise, as I did. My skills developed as I practised because of the supervision I received. The literature is beginning to demonstrate the value of clinical supervision (Swain, 1995), although as with many aspects of nursing, the theory is very different from the practice. Rather than just talking about the benefits of clinical supervision, I want to demonstrate its merits, and I am still striving today to get formal supervision systems in place for all nursing staff within the Trust in which I work. I think too that preparation for supervisory roles needs to be put in place, and that all individuals holding supervisory positions, at managerial or clinical level, should receive training in group dynamics.

I decided to staff in psychiatry for a year to consolidate my training, and worked in a behaviour modification ward. It was wonderful to see seriously disabled individuals rehabilitated into a normal life style back in their own homes. I was able to do more of this work as a community psychiatric nurse (CPN); I worked in this role for almost 5 years. As time went by, I became increasingly intrigued by the different presentations of mental illness and the various approaches available to help people recover from mental illness. The training to become a psychiatric nurse was only 18 months long and although the training gave me an RMN (Registered Mental Nurse) qualification, I realised that it only gave me a basic preparation for practice. Most people did not present with textbook symptoms, and I found that I developed by acquiring skills and up-dating knowledge to meet current needs.

After my initial psychiatric nurse training, in my clinical roles for example, I learned about cognitive therapy and socio-emotional approaches to the care of schizophrenics. I gradually came to the realisation that recovery is possible by tailoring these approaches and skills to the individual patient's needs, understanding of which is obtained by developing relationships with patients and carers. The wisdom of the latter point has been confirmed by the work of Peplau, whose views I have respected over many years; I heard her talk in 1993 and, in her eighties now, she is still inspiring psychiatric nurses (Peplau, 1988).

Autonomous practitioner

I did not return to general nursing. Perhaps I was beginning to see the benefits of investing time and energy into helping patients and carers over a long period of time. I definitely felt that the 'Cinderella' services needed to be fought for, and I think I was inspired by the idea of remaining in psychiatry and developing services which have been ill-provided for. I liked the independence of working in the community where I could manage my own caseload and make decisions about admissions, discharges and the therapeutic input. I felt accountable for my actions and was able to use my clinical skills. The responsibility and solitary nature of the work appealed, and I liked caring for patients in their own homes, where I could involve families. Sinclair (1987) showed that degree nurses tend to be attracted to work in community settings – the degree course may have prepared me well to cope with the more stressful work situations that arise from working on one's own.

Speaking up for the profession

As a CPN, I was able to develop my practice as an autonomous practitioner, and work closely with GPs and the wider primary care team. I became active in the Community Psychiatric Nurses Association and the Scottish Psychiatric Nurses Association. Working within these organisations made me realise how important networking is for development of the individual and the profession. It is crucial too, that organisations like these influence policies and exert pressures at a political level to ensure that nursing developments cater for the needs of the chronically sick as well as those requiring acute, high-tech care. As nurses in the UK, we are lucky to have the needs of nurses represented professionally and nationally, via bodies like the Royal College of Nursing and the UKCC. Nurses are the key professionals who care for patients 24 hours per day; we are thus in a unique position to have an accurate view of patients' needs and the services they require in both hospital and community settings. As managers, educationalists and practitioners, we should take full advantage of these opportunities, and encourage nurses to voice their views and speak up on professional issues.

Power to influence

What kept me in psychiatry was seeing the changes that I was able to make in the lives of my patients and/or carers. Of course, not all patients became well, but I always felt that I was able to help maintain a quality of life for patients that they would not otherwise have had. The ability to change situations for the better is a key factor for me and affects everything I do.

I said earlier that the university course had encouraged me to question and challenge existing practices. In the late 1970s and early 1980s, I must have been the bane of my managers' lives. I was continually pushing them to develop psychiatry in the community. The research evidence from America was showing that short periods in hospital and care at home during a crisis period was effective (Morrice, 1976) and should be developed as an alternative to hospital psychiatry. But it seemed to me that the development of community care, in the UK, was more rhetoric than reality. My managers said that community care, and community psychiatric nursing in particular, were unlikely to expand unless it could be demonstrated that community psychiatric nursing was effective.

Moving on and into research

Understanding 'evaluative' research

Intent on demonstrating such effectiveness, I decided to undertake research into community psychiatric nursing. I applied for and obtained a

Research Training Fellowship from the Scottish Home and Health Department. This enabled me to conduct a study into community psychiatric nursing under the supervision of Susan Sladden, again at Edinburgh University in the Department of Nursing Studies, but this time at the Nursing Research Unit. In many ways this was a wonderful opportunity to learn to do research properly, and to study intensively a topic that I was immensely interested in. I had the idea that I would do my study and come up with proof that community psychiatric nursing was effective. I fantasised that I would present my managers with the results of the study, and lo and behold community psychiatric nursing would be developed! The reality was a little bit different. Like most studies, my research didn't come up with definitive answers to my questions. CPNs were helpful in some ways but not others, and questions remained about how their input differed from that of other professionals.

Acquiring research skills was a first step towards moving away from clinical practice. I definitely learned how to do research, and gained experience and confidence in qualitative and quantitative research methods, in literature searching and information retrieval, in writing and critical appraisal, and in the use of computers. I studied for a doctorate and it was a luxury having time off clinical work to acquire those skills and gain abilities to an advanced level. I learned about evaluative research studies and gained an understanding of effectiveness and efficiency issues, at a time when such matters were highly topical at a policy making level.

Valuing the 'research process' for nurses in practice

Many of the steps in the research process require skills that charge nurses are beginning to develop. Being able to search the literature enables nurses to prepare reports well and keep up-to-date by using libraries, and helps them to undertake the teaching roles required of them. Audit is being integrated increasingly into the work of practising nurses. Audit uses research methods, and computer-held record systems are being introduced into the daily work of nurses. The initial training of nurses needs to embrace these changes and ensure that new staff nurses are prepared and have a basic grasp of research, audit and computer skills.

Becoming self-disciplined

Doing research, however, was incredibly lonely. I'll never forget my first day, walking into the Nursing Research Unit and being shown my room (shared with three others, and being painted at the time, therefore unusable as a base). And that was it – no induction course, no orientation to 'doing research', no introduction whatsoever to place or colleagues. I was just left to get on with it. A far cry from the teamwork I'd been used to as a CPN in the acute admission ward.

Doing research, you have to create your own timetable and demands, set your own deadlines, and meet them. You also have to develop your own supports and relationships, and a confidence in decision making such that you draw your own conclusions about the material you have been reading. Your supervisor is a crucial guide to you, by criticising and giving feedback on your ideas and findings. The rigour of my research is testimony to my research supervisor, Susan Sladden. I am also indebted to Kath Melia who helped me with the qualitative analysis. Both of them contributed positively to my research, but I saw them undertaking roles that were not for me. I need the stimulation and contact with more people than university jobs can offer. I also need to be engaged and involved with projects where I can see more instant and more positive results. However, throughout this period, I did learn to justify and defend decisions, and became self-disciplined in my work.

Moving on and into teaching

In 1985, when I returned to the hospital that had seconded me, the nursing director said that I'd been 'out of service' for so long that I should shadow another charge nurse. I voted with my feet, and rather than shadow a colleague, instead looked for another job – a joint teaching and management (nursing officer) job in a small psychiatric hospital. I was disappointed that the results of my research study were not used to influence CPN practice and was also sorry that I was not able to share my new skills. It is heartening to know that the situation is beginning to change and nursing is slowly but surely becoming more research-orientated (Mullhall, 1995; Pearcey, 1995). An over-riding lesson of that time away from practice is that I believe that training should be followed-up by consolidation in the practice setting. Thankfully, this is happening.

The joint post was for 2 years. I really enjoyed the work, and was told that I 'turned around a culture' of a rural psychiatric hospital. What I know I did was to develop in-service programmes for a wide range of nursing staff, trained and untrained, on both day and night duty. Simultaneously, I gained management experience in the hospital. The job helped me realise how important it is to listen to staff about their perceptions, and to use these views to help them develop their own practice. I enjoyed taking an experiential approach to teaching, using videos and getting staff to do role play – I'm sure it was a powerful means of getting individuals to change their way of working. The downside of a teaching role for me was that I got incredibly nervous and anxious before each teaching session. This, combined with the monotony of repeatedly teaching the same topics every year, would deter me from a teaching career.

Moving on and into nursing management

Motivating staff

I enjoyed the management component of the joint post tremendously. I gradually realised that it was the manager's role to develop opportunities for staff, and to create, not only a learning climate for staff, but also a therapeutic *milieu* for patients. The myth about the manager's role is that it is all administration and form filling. My first job in that joint post disproved that. Yes, there was a certain amount of form filling, but isn't there in all jobs? The nursing officer's role demanded that records be kept of annual leave, sickness and absence, or to confirm shifts worked, for pay purposes; all necessary documentation, which formed a minimal part of the job. Far more of the role consisted of arguing in meetings for resources or systems to be changed, and I could spend as much time as I wanted developing opportunities for staff and supporting them in their endeavours. As a middle manager, I was able to get to know staff and to try and create a system that allowed them to set and achieve high standards. Thus they would be motivated rather than the opposite.

Actions speak louder than words

After the joint nursing officer role, I had a period of 6 months acting up into a managerial job full time. This opportunity made me realise that, of all the roles I had carried out, this was what I wanted to do more of. It seemed to me that this was the role where one could have the most influence and create opportunities to integrate research with practice, decide about roles and job descriptions, have the freedom to develop posts and job-share roles, and ensure that orientation and teaching programmes were followed through at ward level, or that clinical supervision systems are put into place ... the list is endless. I also came to realise that it isn't only the positive actions which carry weight. Identifying the poor performer or bad practice and changing behaviour to the acceptable, or making unpopular decisions and justifying actions fairly and openly, were equally important in showing by actions that, as a manager, I believed that quality of care is important. Adair (1991) and Clutterbuck *et al.* (1992) confirm my views of leadership and managing. To obtain a management role was to be my next challenge.

Open and consistent approach

I found it difficult to obtain a line management post. Until I did, I worked directly with the director of nursing services on manpower planning and on clinical grading. This latter was a nationally-driven exercise in re-grading nursing posts (Gavin, 1995). The designers of the grades obviously did not have a research background, as they did not operationalise their definitions. Clinical grading was a very negative experience for me, and demonstrated how badly and unsystematically nursing had been managed in the past. I vowed that if I was ever in a management post in the future, I would try to be consistent and systematic in my decision making. Clinical grading provided me with the opportunity to work with senior management within the hospital setting and at Board level. I gained an insight into formal grievance procedures and the systems used nationally to deal with them.

Positive in the face of criticism

My first three applications for line management posts were unsuccessful. The interview feedback I received stated that they'd been impressed with me but that I lacked management experience. Traditional experience indeed I may have lacked, but I would argue that I had alternative experiences that would hold me in good stead for any management role. My research experience, which I described earlier, meant that I had acquired skills in time management and meeting deadlines, important in relation to report writing and project work. I learned from the experience of working alone, drawing on my own resources, and being able to continue to work positively in the face of criticism and negative feedback – excellent preparation for a management role, I would argue. There was also an indication that the interviewers thought that I would not stay in a management role, and they expressed the view that I was 'academic' material (whatever that means).

My arguments about the skills I had to offer (from my unique experience) fell on deaf ears, until I was successful in obtaining a director of nursing services post in the north of Scotland. What an opportunity! As one of the most highly graded DNS posts in Scotland, it not only presented a major challenge in management terms, but also provided experience of commissioning the building of a new psychiatric hospital and, in parallel, expanding community care. The 4 years I spent away from the comfort of my training area were a wonderful challenge and offered tremendously exciting development opportunities for me. I recommend that staff move away from their parent training areas, if they are serious about developing a career in nursing. Such a move allows skills to be tested and abilities developed in an arena where your previous track record and 'novice' status are unknown.

Managing change and involving staff

Grampian Health Board, under the direction of Hance Fullerton, took organisational change and development seriously (Fullerton *et al.*, 1989). A random 10% of staff were surveyed, every 2 years, to ascertain what improvements needed to take place, and to measure the impact of change generally. I was impressed with the systematic approach that was taken to getting staff involved in the change process. The surveys obtained staff views about what had to be done better and what had to be dealt with by the senior managers. Thus staff had the power to influence change in a major way. The whole approach was a sterling attempt to reduce the 'us and them' divide that separates the workforce from those that manage them. I am proud to have been involved in that attempt.

Change agents were introduced after the first survey, as was team briefing to improve communications. The change agents actively developed teamwork in local situations. After the second survey, a major training exercise was mounted to develop supervisors and equip them with skills and tools to help them manage well. Some say that it takes 8–12 years to change a culture (Plant, 1987), and many staff were sceptical about the organisational development approach that was being used. Having come from working in an area in which this approach was not taken, I could see the benefits of getting staff involved. The disadvantage was that increasing staff awareness of what was going on could make some staff suspicious and anxious about the changes that were happening.

Creating a mental health strategy: the big picture

One of the first tasks I was involved in as the director of nursing services was to contribute to the mental health strategy. Nursing developments within the community were high profile. The strategy was developed within 6 months by all the key professionals and voluntary groups getting together and documenting what they wanted to see happening for psychiatry in the next 10 years. It was exciting working with the key players and creating a joint vision of what we wanted to see develop over the next few years. The Specific Grant for Mental Illness and Bridging Finance, made available by the government as pump priming, made it possible for the vision to become a reality, and joint work could make it possible. Psychiatric nurses in the community were crucial to making the vision work.

Developing roles for psychiatric nurses

Most senior managers begin with restructuring the systems in which they work. I was no different and I revised the structures on day and night duty. I organised development workshops for the nursing officers so that they could explore and clearly understand their role in the monitoring and maintenance of standards within psychiatric nursing. The number of nurse managers was reduced, and the importance of the charge nurse's role at ward level re-affirmed. The day duty charge nurses assumed 24-hour responsibility, and, in tandem, primary nursing was widely introduced at ward level. Specialist posts in community nursing and rehabilitation were created to underline the expertise of psychiatric nurses and make prominent the skills and valuable contribution that psychiatric nursing can make. As line manager of all the nurses in the psychiatric speciality, I made the above changes which were discussed and agreed by the general manager and the medical superintendent. The structure made professional leadership possible.

Moving on and into general management

Planning community developments

The NHS Management Enquiry (HMSO, 1983) introduced general management into the NHS, and the NHS reforms, driven by central policy (Department of Health, 1989a), resulted in nursing becoming decreasingly managed by nurses. In Grampian, general management was fully introduced in 1991 and the director of nursing services role I had occupied disappeared. I then became general manager of four hospitals in Grampian, and had special responsibility for the development of community psychiatry. I was saddened not to be able to see through and push for further developments within psychiatric nursing, but it was exciting to be at the forefront of community care.

There was a really good joint planning structure in Grampian, involving health, social work, housing, education and the voluntary organisations. I was a member of each of the four planning groups and helped put in place plans to develop facilities for the psychiatrically ill. Care management pilots were set up (Department of Health, 1989b), and mental health teams (Patmore & Weaver, 1991) started. I set the ball rolling for one of the old psychiatric hospitals to be closed, and developed quality standards for the re-location of 30 demented patients into a private setting. I produced a monthly brief about the changes, and had routine meetings with staff – a daunting forum where what I was doing was questioned and challenged by staff.

Such regular, face-to-face contact is crucial in a period of major change, and I believe that all managers should develop some sort of routine whereby they have a dialogue with staff and provide opportunities for staff to talk through and gain an understanding of planning priorities. This is important as the National Health Service is becoming more 'business oriented' given the 'market philosophy' of current government policy (Bradshaw, 1995).

Juggling study and work

Partly because of the business emphasis within the NHS, I decided to do a part-time business degree. I wanted to understand more about the dynamics within commercial enterprises. It was obvious that 'outsiders', with business experience, were gaining senior positions within the NHS, and I wanted to equip myself with some of the know-how and acumen that they had. The first term of the business degree (MBA) was the only time in my life that I have felt stressed. Monday and Wednesday nights were lectures on accountancy and managerial economics respectively. I enjoyed the latter, although dredging up calculus and quadratic equations from school days to do some of the forecasting exercises was quite a shock to the system. The accountancy was a nightmare and to this day I will shy away from anything that even hints at dual entry book-keeping.

What was horrific about that first term was not the subjects I was confronted with, but rather the pressure of studying two completely new topics from scratch, to degree level. It meant working at the weekends, and studying and doing essays and assignments in addition to the pressures of a demanding job. I decided only to do one subject per term. That meant I did the degree in 3 years instead of 2, an achievement that I am really proud of. To study part-time and work is not easy. You need to be committed and determined in order to make time to study. You also need good friends and family to keep the studying in perspective and keep a good balance of work and pleasure.

Understanding the business world

I studied all sorts of subjects that were foreign to me – strategic planning, marketing, operational management, organisational behaviour – and gained new insights into running businesses. The students on the course were all senior managers within their respective firms. Contact with them made me realise how complex the National Health Service is, and gave me confidence in my managerial role. I was now able to express what we were doing in the National Health Service, in business terms. I now understand more than just nursing, can question other specialists, e.g. strategic planners and accountants, and am in a better position to ensure that the reason for the existence of the National Health Service – caring for patients – does not get lost amongst the interests of marketing, cost containment, business planning and the balance sheet.

Promoting a quality improvement culture

My third and final job in Grampian was as director of quality, a senior management post, the aim of which was to develop quality within the Trust. I organised a small, centralised department consisting of nine people. We began by developing a strategy and operational plan for quality development. To produce this, I had to read a lot about 'quality'. And again, this opportunity was invaluable.

In 'business management' the notion of 'quality' has been around for years and numerous books have been written by individuals who have become known as 'quality gurus' – people like Deming, Crosbie, Juran, Oakland and Donabedian (see Oakland,1990; and Department of Trade and Industry, 1992, 1993, for summary texts). These authors produced concepts like 'total quality management', 'quality control' and 'quality assurance', and developed techniques like brainstorming, quality circles and measurement approaches as useful tools and means of presentation for managers. Definitions like 'fit for purpose', 'striving for excellence', 'zero defect rate' and 'continuous improvement' have emerged from their writings and have begun to slip into the jargon of policy and planning documents (Wilson Report, 1994; Audit Commission, 1992).

Many staff are resistant to the TQM (total quality management) programmes which are being introduced within the National Health Service. Nevertheless, books on the topic of 'quality' have been produced as texts specifically for health service staff (see Wilson, 1992; Ovretveit, 1992) and for nurses (see Bull, 1992; Parsley & Corrigan, 1994; Marr & Giebing, 1994). Course curricula need to be modified to include 'quality improvement' for nursing staff. Ideally sessions like these should be multi-disciplinary to facilitate inter-agency and inter-professional debate about working together to produce quality systems and processes. Given that such training has not previously existed, staff can be antagonistic towards the introduction of 'new' initiatives like TQM which can be seen as implying that quality has not previously existed. This of course is quite wrong, but what the National Health Service needs to do better is to reduce wastage and promote inter-departmental working and teamwork to tackle problems at the root and prevent recurrence of difficulties. Only then will we be an efficient and effective organisation.

Becoming efficient and effective

We have been very good, as professionals, at talking about the value of the NHS. We must start to measure and quantify what we are doing. This exercise, only really beginning, has been driven by the government's reforms, aimed at reducing public spending. I firmly believe that we cannot examine activity and costs without looking at the quality of the service we are providing, and over the next few years we must produce evidence of the benefits of the care that we currently provide. This is a challenge which demands involvement of all staff together, not just managers. We need to strive to work together so that individuals are motivated to achieve high standards, minimise complaints and reduce wastage to nil. We are quite a way from achieving those goals, but I would like to see them attained before I retire.

Moving back to psychiatric nursing

Professional advisory role

I left Grampian in 1993 and returned to a post in Lothian, as director of nursing and quality. The difference between this post and my original Grampian director of nursing services post was that the new role did not involve line management over nurses. The director plays a strategic role and advises the chief executive (and others) about professional develop-ments and requirements. In some ways it is frustrating to be advising rather than implementing, because I am left in a position of troubleshooting and intervening after situations have reached crisis point, rather than preventing crises. The changes I wish to influence in nursing happen more slowly, too, because I am not in a position to steer the pace and quality of their introduction. The main forum through which I effect change is via a monthly meeting with senior nurses from each service area. It is here that issues like UKCC requirements are debated and professional matters like clinical supervision or the implications of the Allitt Inquiry (HMSO, 1994) are taken forward.

Integration of research, audit and development

After a year, I relinquished the 'quality' element of the role, as we decided not to have a central approach to the development of quality, but rather, under the direction of the chief executive, to let each service manager take the quality drive forward. I am very happy with this and think it is up to each and every one of us to create a climate in which quality is well and truly on the map. Having relinquished the quality role, I was asked to take on the community general manager's role in addition to the nursing director's role. I couldn't have a more perfect role, and I love (almost) every minute of this job because, as the line manager of the community service, I can influence directly the development of community care within the Trust. To date, I have (of course) restructured the community set-up and created new posts in research and audit.

I would like to make research-based practice a reality within the community service and integrate audit with daily practice as suggested by recent policy documents (SHHD, 1993, 1994). I have taken beginning steps in this direction. I have already supervised one research project in psychiatry which looked at the learning climate and joint working relationships between the service area and the local nursing college (Forrest & Brown, 1994). I will continue to undertake supervision with identified individuals and support nurses to do small research projects within their normal work. Their research work is motivated by an enthusiasm to improve services and I am sure that it is done over and above their normal working day. I do try, however, to encourage other nurses with research skills to seek funding for research. This enables me to replace staff and release nurses to do the much needed research and audit work.

With a university colleague, I have recently obtained a research grant to evaluate CPNs' care of people with enduring mental illness. I have just submitted a proposal to audit the care of patients receiving long-term depot medication; this project will audit whether the standards of practice identified by the RCN (1994) are being put into place and will build on the work of Turner (1994).

All of the above examples illustrate how research and audit are being put into practice. It is exciting that the climate is now right to do this, given the need to evaluate and measure the effect of our endeavours. We are seeing an increasing emphasis in psychiatry and mental health on highlighting outcome indicators of services being set up (Jenkins, 1990; Dean, 1994). We are being required to 'benchmark' our services and demonstrate, by comparison, that our services reflect good practice (see Zaire & Hutton, 1995; Hollings, 1992). This 'benchmarking' must result in the development of services to benefit patients and carers.

One of the advantages of being in a strategic role is having the ability to create roles, and to control my work so that I can influence the direction of the service. A good recent example of this is the work that I've done with colleagues, including GPs, to develop a community mental health team (CMHT). This latter project is designed to compare and contrast the working of the CMHT with two other services, a GP-attached CPN, and the traditional, existing hospital-attached CPNs. Hopefully, this project will provide data for the purchaser to develop future services, and the CMHT project is evidence of the benefit of improved joint working with GPs.

These examples again demonstrate how research is being integrated into practice, and demonstrate that R & D is here to stay (SHHD 1993). These examples are also evidence that there is support to develop community care and a desire to develop future services provision based on good practice and tried and tested models of delivery.

Conclusion

Given this review of my career, you can be forgiven for thinking that I am a certificate collector. However, my collection of degrees has almost been co-incidental. What has driven me has been a desire for knowledge and understanding to enable me to lead well, and to direct service developments which are judged to be of a high standard. I do not miss practical nursing, as I feel that in my current role, albeit in a different way, I influence the development of psychiatric nursing by supporting and facilitating good practice, and by creating opportunities for innovation and quality care provision.

As a psychiatric nurse, I had to make the decision to move into 'management' roles. This decision in a way closed doors to a teaching or academic career, and meant that I have left practical nursing and direct patient care behind me. I do not regret this decision at all. I am able to focus all my energy on the management tasks, and on strategic and operational planning. Doctors in management roles, e.g. clinical directors and the medical directors of Trusts, combine clinical and managerial roles. They assert that in order to do a 'good' management job they have to retain clinical work. I have had combined roles myself and I disagree with their assertion. Joint roles result in compromises and detract from the post-holder's ability to function fully in any one role. The NHS reforms, and particularly the introduction of clinical directorates (Barker, 1990), offer advantages in terms of developing multi-disciplinary care for specific groups of patients. Clinical directorates have succeeded in getting medical staff involved and participating in management roles within the health service. This is a first step, but I believe that doctors will never be able to engage totally in management roles until some doctors decide to assume such posts full-time.

In my review, I have tried to illustrate how I have moved into and within psychiatric nursing. Changes arising from the NHS reforms have meant that I have had several roles which have taken me away from psychiatric nursing itself. Many, though not all, of the reforms are creating a better health service. I recently read the following: 'I deplore the fashionable tendency to focus on problems rather than opportunities, to belittle what we do well and concentrate instead on what we do badly, to ignore the tremendous advances we have seen in our lifetime, and to indulge in pessimistic guesswork' (Davis, 1995). These words echo my sentiments entirely and portray accurately a culture which has traditionally pervaded (psychiatric) nursing.

I consciously try to bring to my work a positive view of the NHS changes, and to counteract the negative perspective that pervades our work environment. Even in my short career, psychiatric nursing has made tremendous strides and developments are happening today, e.g. in research and development and in community care, which were inconceivable in the 1980s. I'm sure that the next decade will be equally productive, and that progress will continue. The drive to develop community care is here to stay, as is the imperative to develop performance and outcome measures (Payne, 1994). I enjoy being in a position to influence developments positively in the direction of these policies which, as this account shows, are of special interest to me.

I have not planned my career from the outset. Many of the opportunities presented by accident. I have perhaps been in the right place at the right time – I don't know. What I do know is that I have made the best of situations and have consciously driven myself to 'make things happen' rather than be a passive recipient of change. I have taken full advantage of being one of the 'lucky generation' described by Davis (1995). You are too, and as a closing comment, I recommend this text to you.

References

Adair, J. (1991) *Not Bosses but Leaders*. Kogan Page, London.

Audit Commission (1992) *The Virtue of Patients: Making Best Use of Ward Nursing Resources*, 2nd edn. HMSO, London.

Barker, P. (1990) The Leicester experience. *The Health Service Journal* **100**, 1428–1429.

Bentley, H. (1996) The need for change in nurse education: a literature review. *Health Education Today* **16**, 131–136.

Bradshaw, P.L. (1995) The recent health reforms in the United Kingdom: some tentative observations on their impact on nurses and nursing in hospitals. *Journal of Advanced Nursing* **21**, 975–979.

Buchan, J., Ball, J. & Thomas, S. (1993) *The 'Effective' Ward Sister – A Review of the Literature*. CSO, Edinburgh.

Bull, N. (1992) *Quality: For Those Who Care*. Information Press, Oxford.

Clutterbuck, D., Dearlove, D. & Snow, D. (1992) *Actions Speak Louder. A Management Guide to Corporate Social Responsibility*. Kogan Page, London.

Davis, W. (1995) *The Lucky Generation: A Positive View of the 21st Century*. Headline Books, London.

Dean, C. (1994) *A Slow Train Coming. Bringing the Mental Health Revolution to Scotland*. Greater Glasgow Community Mental Health Services NHS Trust, Glasgow.

Department of Health (1989a) *Working for Patients*. HMSO, London.

Department of Health (1989b) *Caring for People: Community Care in the Next Decade and Beyond*. HMSO, London.

Department of Trade and Industry (1992) *The Quality Gurus: What Can They do for Your Company?* 2nd edn. Department of Trade and Industry, London.

Department of Trade and Industry (1993) *Total Quality Management and Effective Leadership: A Strategic Overview*, 2nd edn. Department of Trade and Industry, London.

Forrest, S. & Brown, N. (1994) *The Clinical Role of the Nurse Teacher: An Exploratory Study of Perceptions of the Nurse Teacher's Present and Ideal Role in the Clinical Area*. Lothian College of Health Studies, Edinburgh.

Fullerton, H., Ironside, A. & Price, C. (1989) A picture of health in the 1990s. *The Health Service Journal* **99**, 730–732.

Gavin, J.H. (1995) The politics of nursing: a case study – clinical grading. *Journal of Advanced Nursing* **22**, 378–385.

Goffman, E. (1975) *Asylums. Essays on the Social Situation of Mental Patients and Other Inmates* 5th edn. Pelican, London.

Hallet, C.E., Hillier, V.F., Orr, J.A. & Butterworth, T. (1995) The time commitment of the community nursing services to Project 2000. *Journal of Advanced Nursing* **15** (4), 250–256.

HMSO (1983) *NHS Management Enquiry*. HMSO, London.

HMSO (1994) *The Allitt Inquiry. Independent Inquiry Relating to Deaths and Injuries on the Children's Ward at Grantham and Kesteven General Hospital During the Period February to April*. HMSO, London.

Hollings, L. (1992) Clearing up the confusion about benchmarking. *The TQM Magazine*. **4** (3), 149–151.

Jenkins, R. (1990) Towards a system of outcome indicators in mental health. *British Journal of Psychiatry* **157**, 500–514.

Kreitman, N., Smith, P., Gries, S. *et al*. (1969) Parasuicide. *British Journal of Psychiatry* **115**, 746–747.

Lemmer, B. & Smits, M. (1989) *Facilitating Change in Mental Health*. Chapman and Hall, London.

Manning, N. (1989) *The Therapeutic Community Movement: Charisma and Routinization*. Routledge, London.

Marr, H. & Giebing, H. (1994) *Quality Assurance in Nursing. Concepts, Methods and Case Studies*. Campion Press, Edinburgh.

Martin, J.P. (1984) *Hospitals in Trouble*. Blackwell Science, Oxford.

Menzies, I.E.P. (1960) A case study in the functioning of social systems as a defence against anxiety. *Human Relations* **13**, 95–121.

Morrice, J.K.W. (1976) *Crisis Intervention: Studies in Community Care*. Pergamon Press, Oxford.

Mullhall, A. (1995) Nursing research – what difference does it make? *Journal of Advanced Nursing* **21** (3), 576–583.

Oakland, J.S. (1990) *Total Quality Management*. Butterworth–Heinemann, London.

Ovretveit, J. (1992) *Health Service Quality: An Introduction to Quality Methods for Health Services*. Blackwell Science, Oxford.

Parsley, K. & Corrigan, P. (1994) *Quality Improvement in Nursing and Healthcare. A Practical Approach*. Chapman and Hall, London.

Patmore, C. & Weaver, T. (1991) *Community Mental Health Teams: Lessons for Planners and Managers*. Good Practices in Mental Health, London.

Payne, R. (1994) *Outcome Measurement in Community Care*. Community Care Implementation Unit, Edinburgh.

Pearcey, P.A. (1995) Achieving research-based practice. *Journal of Advanced Nursing* **22**, 33–39.

Peplau, H. (1988) *Interpersonal Relations in Nursing*. Macmillan Education, London.

Plant, R. (1987) *Managing Change and Making it Stick*. William Collins and Sons, Glasgow.

RCN (1994) *Good Practice in the Administration of Depot Neuroleptics. A Guidance Document for Mental Health and Practice Nurses*. Department of Health, London.

SHHD (1993) *Research and Development Strategy for NHS in Scotland*. Chief Scientist's Office, Edinburgh.

SHHD (1994) *Moving to Audit: An Education Package for Nurses, Midwives and Health Visitors*. University of Dundee Centre for Medical Education and CRAG, Dundee.

Sinclair, H.C. (1987) Graduate nurses in the United Kingdom: myth and reality. *Nurse Education Today* **7**, 24–29.

Swain, G. (1995) *Clinical Supervision: The Principles and Process*. Health Visitors Association, London.

Turner, G.N. (1994) Organisational climate and standards of nursing care: the administration of depot neuroleptic drugs to psychiatric out-patients. PhD thesis, Edinburgh University, Edinburgh.

White, E. (1995) Project 2000: the early experience of mental health nurses. In *Community Psychiatric Nursing* (C. Brooker & E. White eds). Chapman and Hall, London, pp. 95–115.

Wilson, C.R.M. (1992) *Strategies in Health Care Quality*. WB Saunders, London.

Wilson Report (1994) *Being Heard: The Report of a Review Committee in NHS Complaints Procedures*. Department of Health, Edinburgh.

Zaire, M. & Hutton, R. (1995) Benchmarking, a process-driven tool for quality improvement. *The TQM Magazine* **7** (3), 35–40.

7 Taking Stock of Psychiatric Nursing

Susan Ritter

Introduction

Whether there is a system of mental or psychiatric or mental health nursing is doubtful. Rather there are sets of beliefs held by psychiatric nurses who are constrained by the statutory frameworks of the Nurses, Midwives and Health Visitors Acts and Rules, the Mental Health Act 1983 and associated legislation. To be able to act as a system, what is currently known as mental health nursing must be able to point to beliefs and goals that cohere with its actions. If there ever was a consensus about psychiatric nursing it finally vanished in the incoherence and paradoxes of restricted access to medical help in a health service driven by a rhetoric of choice and excellence.

In this chapter I consider many aspects of the contradictory dogmas, ideologies and ambiguities that trouble psychiatric nursing. I assume that the purpose of psychiatric nursing is mediation, defined as the management of ambiguity. I argue that nursing in the United Kingdom is part of a health service, fragmented though it is, and needs to exist within an academic framework that integrates in a credible fashion the spectrum of health services studies. I suggest that our over-indulgence in pseudo-philosophy has contributed to our position at the bottom of the league table of disciplines in the 1996 Research Assessment Exercise.

I explore putative legitimating frameworks for psychiatric nursing practice, beginning with ultimately unsuccessful moral justifications for nurses' actions, moving on to discuss various accounts given by nurses of their practice. I argue that in the 1970s and 1980s the education and training of psychiatric nurses combined three incompatible ways of accounting for practice. I identify contradictions in the way that nursing knowledge embodies practical rather than theoretical reasoning, while the profession values research that is removed from everyday practice. I suggest that the problems of psychiatric nurse training have disconnected it from recent developments in education as a whole.

I suggest that in an attempt to break out of the loop of unsubstantiated practice, unsubstantiated education and fragmentary knowledge base, psychiatric nurses have evolved ineffective strategies which reflect the ambiguities and contradictions already inherent in nursing practice, and which are put to bad use in order to avoid tackling these unpalatable issues. Although the nursing profession is no less a mirror of prevailing social structures than the medical profession, these strategies make it difficult for psychiatric nurses to collaborate with other professions and disciplines. I argue that while nursing's move to institutions of higher education has contributed to the tightening of the grip of a libertarian/authoritarian clerisy in psychiatric nursing, users of psychiatric nurses' services now have access to information and other resources that enable them to influence mental health care without the need for nurses to act as brokers.

I argue that enforcement is as likely an outcome of nurses' actions as enabling, and to that end I consider in detail aspects of the lexicon of psychiatric nurses. Nurses believe that many of their actions must be cloaked in objectivity, hence their professional caution in reporting on what they do, shown in their discourse, in their records and in talk about patients. I argue that elements of nurses' discourse (both in its restricted sense of written and spoken prose and its wider sense that includes praxis) contradict ostensible beliefs in theories of demystification. I describe my experience of a clinical experiment that failed, in order to reconsider and extend my discussion of diagnosis. I suggest that if the therapeutic relationship is a set of interactional practices, some of which are ambiguous, then nurses become doubtful about who is a victim of so-called psychiatric power. I argue that nurses have been actively complicit in the creation of managed competition and in the savings in employment costs that competitive health care necessitates.

Having cast much of my argument in terms of disconnection, removal from, fragmentation, contradiction and ambiguity, I return to the theme of mediation. I redefine the purpose of mediation in order to explore alternative ways of accounting for psychiatric nursing practice, and of organising programmes of education and training. I finish the chapter by hoping that it is possible for psychiatric nurses to join a new cross-sectional alliance between the mental health and social services and their patients, clients and users.

The purpose of psychiatric nursing

Jenny Littlewood (1991, p. 185) hypothesises that 'caring, the nurse's central role, is the management of ambiguity'. I understand her to be arguing that this management consists of mediating between internal and external worlds. Because she is writing about hospital nursing she describes mediation in terms of helping patients to manage their bodies, especially their faeces, vomit and blood, thus maintaining the boundaries between self and the outside world. As with any anecdote, different people have different experiences (see Evans, 1995), but my recent experiences as a carer indicate that increasingly control of what Littlewood calls 'body marginals' may be handed over in hospital to the patient or to unqualified staff. I have seen post-operative patients helplessly vomiting unobserved by nurses until alerted by a visitor or another patient, when a health care assistant or Project 2000 student is sent with a bowl, and I have changed bloody sheets myself. In the community, care may be handed over to female relations, female neighbours, female friends – any woman who will lessen the workload of the district nurse. In other words nurses, instead of mediating directly between patients and the consequences of their illness, mediate between a variety of support staff and other professionals.

In psychiatry the nurse is no less a mediator between internal and external worlds, but the nurse infers and maintains the boundaries of the internal world of a patient through interpretation of what he or she hears and sees. The nurse's interpretation may help to modulate the counter-active tensions of the patient's ambiguous relationship with the outside world, or it may not. If mediation is the purpose of nursing then Gillian Rose's (1992) reminder of its etymology in what she calls the 'broken middle' hints at a key theme. Mediation does not aim to mend, resolve or correct, but to hold in suspension opposing forces. However, as in general nursing, there is evidence that psychiatric nurses are increasingly med-iating between patients and services or agencies, rather than directly between patients and the consequences of their illness.

Psychiatric nursing in higher education

In the mid-1990s the Tomlinson and Culyer reports shook up the teaching hospitals and their associated medical schools in London with the result that funding for research and development in the National Health Service was tied ever more closely to existing achievements in research. In the week that I was finishing this chapter the results of the 1996 United Kingdom research assessment exercise were published. Despite high scores for two or three departments, nursing as a discipline finished last in the league table, its weighted average nearly one point below the penul-timate discipline, professions allied to medicine, and very little changed over the previous 15 years.

Perhaps professional departments (focusing on vocational education) to a great extent exclude research opportunities, and there are grounds for arguing that these ways of managing research are at base a procedure for minimising expenditure, effectively excluding certain kinds of research, although English and Philosophy finished above nursing in the league tables. I am lucky to work in a multi-faculty environment where there are research opportunities and resources for staff who wish to do higher degrees. This inevitably shapes my view that rather than competing with other disciplines, especially medicine, nursing needs to collaborate, if it is not merely to survive but to have some influence over the future devel-opment of health care.

Legitimating frameworks

Since the early 1970s psychiatric nurses have argued that despite the supporting framework of mental health legislation the power they wield over patients is not legitimate. They have contended that the technology of psychiatry has promoted control and repression of patients. That is, the political underpinnings of psychiatric practice are essentially immoral.

This contention has also served to justify the lack of research into day-to-day psychiatric nursing interventions. If psychiatric nursing is a profession without legitimacy then research into its skills is necessarily illegitimate. Until psychiatric nurses centre their activities in a legitimating moral framework any attempts by them to justify their interventions by research into effectiveness will be worthless. The debate is often cast in the form of attacks on so-called scientific methods and so-called positivist approaches to psychiatry.

Similar arguments may also be used to condone all attempts by nurses to deal with their daily work. They weigh competing moral justifications for their actions in order to feel comfortable with what they do. A kind of utilitarianism often forms such moral justification. For example, if we are short of staff it is the fault of our managers, who are the way they are because of an unjust social system. Because we are short of staff (the social system is unjust) we are unable to deal with patients as we or they would wish and we must be expedient with individuals in order to prevent harm to the majority (harm being defined perhaps as stress to staff, or disruption to other patients). It is immaterial that there is no evidence for the clinical effectiveness of a nurse's actions, it is sufficient that he or she can provide a moral justification (compare 'practical reasoning', discussed later in this chapter).

Psychiatric nurses share a perception that what they do is in the patient's interests even if it means locking someone up who is not detained under the Mental Health Act 1983. Paradoxically, by invoking a utilitarian justification, nurses also shed personal responsibility as moral agents (as Peter Sedgwick (1982) observed of the trade unionists who used to prevent undesirable patients being admitted to wards or hospitals). Such moral sleight-of-hand lies behind many of the difficulties psychiatric nurses have in agreeing about what they do, let alone what they ought to do.

What are a patient's interests, how are they construed by nurses, and how is this affected by the moral obligations that nurses feel towards patients? Psychiatric nurses tend to adopt defensive postures in the face of the 'obligations, rules, norms and values' (Wynne, 1978, p. 186) that comprise professional practice within the mental health services. Wynne argues that the 'rubber fence' moulded by these constraints is a powerful source of contradictory, ambiguous and disqualifying communications both to staff and patients, prefiguring Ruth Gallop's assertion that statutory powers are mostly used to control patients, not as a context for restoring a sense of control to them. The rubber fence becomes a metaphor for the unlawful restraint embodied in the threat to 'section' a patient who does not take his or her medication, and for the restricted reasoning expressed in the fear of the coroner's court. The rubber fence also surrounds psychiatric nurses who adopt (regardless of their gender) paternalistic and confrontational interventions such as control and restraint or seclusion.

With the introduction of the supervision register has come a proliferation of health care workers with legal powers to coerce unwilling patients into treatment. Two opposing risks ensue. One is that making responsive relationships with people in their own homes and negotiating individual care plans are subordinated to controlling disturbed behaviour (itself seen as a specialist intervention). The other is that despite the availability of coercive treatment provisions patients still manage to kill themselves and other people, often to the surprise of the agencies and teams responsible for their care (Steering Group, 1996).

Education and training in the 1970s and 1980s

Many factors maintain the rubber fence. Some of these factors originate in the recent history of psychiatric nursing. Though associated with norms and values, they deprive nurses of theoretical principles for the organisation of their work, for research, and for forming explicit rules for practice in clinical settings. In the late 1970s and early 1980s, still driven by the impetus of earlier work, especially by sociologists of deviance and by ethnomethodologists, nurse educators drafted the 1982 syllabus for training leading to the qualification of registered mental nurse, published by the General Nursing Council very shortly before its separation into the United Kingdom Central Council and the National Boards for Nursing, Midwifery and Health Visiting.

At that time it seemed not only that teleological models were acceptable material for students of nursing to use in their search for understanding of their chosen profession, but also that it was acceptable to yoke together widely disparate sociological approaches in order to construct an image of the psychiatric nurse to which students could aspire. Curricula adopted perspectives ultimately derived from Marx's nineteenth century writing which took the view that the nurse's role should be one of demystification, to act as the patient's agent in achieving freedom from unnecessary social authority whose oppression was exemplified by the labelling processes of psychiatry. Other perspectives on the psychiatric nurse derived from ethnomethodological studies which sought to render faithfully the social lives of mental hospitals.

This literature was highly successful in getting to grips with the everyday life of hospitals (the petty tyranny, the arbitrariness of authority, the collectivisation of nursing care, the 'anonymising' of individuals), but because none of this related to aspirant nurses, lessons from the literature tended to be framed in terms of what to avoid. Leaders were automatically suspect, especially if they were psychiatrists; patients had a right not to get up, not to bathe, not to take medication; uniforms for nurses were done away with; and patients were to be addressed by their first names.

During the same period John Dewey's (1963) philosophy of learning from experience was increasingly systematised in order to make the teaching of group dynamics and psychodynamics manageable. Critical theory as applied to psychiatric nursing demanded that the individual nurse hold an explicitly moral attitude to his or her work. Experiential learning as applied to psychiatric nursing demanded that the individual nurse claim to know only what he or she had experienced. Ethnomethodology (despite its incompatibility with critical theory) demonstrated to the psychiatric nurse the depths to which he or she would descend if personal experience and personal authority were ignored.

A third component of the 1982 syllabus was its emphasis on using the nursing process, whose quasi-scientific approach appeared to be at odds with the other elements. Its emphasis on problem-solving led inevitably to attempts to reify patients' problems, often to attempts to use standardised care plans, and to confusion between clinical staff, who could not see why they should use the nursing process, teaching staff, who rarely applied it clinically, and students, who were trying to make sense of the competing influences of their education (in the classroom) and their training (in clinical settings).

Practical and theoretical reasoning

One effect of a programme comprising such disparate parts is that the link between thought or intention and actions becomes especially problematic because actions which follow premises cannot be true or false (Guttenplan, 1994). This is practical reasoning, as I have seen, for example, in internet nursing discussion groups which argue that nursing knowledge does not need to involve evidence, reason, logic, observation, perception, confirmation or probability: 'Trust me, I'm a nurse'. As Ruth Gallop has observed, in a paper delivered at the 1995 Canadian Federation of Mental Health Nurses/Clarke Institute of Psychiatry conference on Mental Health Care: The Challenge of Change, psychiatric nurses acquire skills by osmosis rather than systematically and the skills that are taught systematically tend to be generic counselling techniques rather than specific interventions. The original purpose of teaching generic counselling techniques like open questioning, echoing and reflection, was to ensure that the patient could disclose and describe inner experiences. Instead counselling has become an end in itself, with the consequence that interviews or conversations simply become directionless (interminable?). As a result, we have no idea what duration, frequency, content or style of contact with nurses is required by people with severe mental illness living at home. In such circumstances, as Lewis Wolpert (1992, p. 134) observes of psychoanalysis, 'what evidence, what experiment, what new data would persuade [them] to change their ideas?'.

Apart from nurse behaviour therapy, there is no organised body of knowledge about the relationship between psychiatric nursing care and specific patient outcomes. Apart from nurse behaviour therapy, there is no demonstrable and consistent use of feedback in order to modify psychiatric nursing care. Apart from nurse behaviour therapy, psychiatric nursing care has not been demonstrated to be effective in clinically replicated studies. Apart from nurse behaviour therapy the success rate of psychiatric nursing care cannot be demonstrated. Apart from nurse behaviour therapy, there is no evidence that one psychiatric nurse practises skills that are directly comparable with the skills of another psychiatric nurse.

Research in itself is not a universal remedy. For many years the concept of nursing research has dominated the thinking of academic nurses. That is, they have emphasised nursing research rather than research into the contribution of nurses to the treatment and care of people with specific disorders such as bipolar disorder or schizophrenia. For an unpublished paper in 1988 I found and classified 205 articles about psychiatric nursing published in the previous 10 years according to the type of study and the subject-matter. I was partly trying to make sense of my experience in writing my first book, *The Bethlem Royal and Maudsley Hospital Manual of Clinical Psychiatric Nursing Principles and Procedures* (Ritter, 1989), which had preoccupied me over the preceding 3 years and for which I had tried to establish a research-based foundation. I used Sills's (1977) categories: research that addresses social systems; research that addresses interpersonal relationships; and research that explores individual or personal issues. The frequencies are shown in Table 7.1.

Table 7.1

Type of study	The system	The relationship	The person	Total
Descriptive	37	37	57	131
Experimental	03	07	01	11
Quasi-experimental	0	01	0	01
Theoretical	28	01	02	31
Literature review	07	02	05	14
Historical	11	0	0	11
Anecdotal	02	04	0	06
Total	88	52	65	205

There appeared to be minimal empirical work. How the research was initiated was not often made clear. There were few hypotheses. The aims and strategy of the research were rarely explicit or linked in any systematic way. It was impossible to make links between studies or to pursue questions, issues and arguments. The most that I could do was, like Grace Sills, to identify themes. Worst of all I could not find studies that were based on clear principles of psychiatric nursing practice. For example, among questions that remained unanswered from the 1960s were whether nurses were in fact able to differentially reinforce behaviour (Ayllon & Azrin, 1964), or whether they could modify symptomatic verbal behaviour of people with schizophrenia (Ayllon & Haughton, 1964). As far as I know they are still unanswered. Coincidentally, Robinson & Elkan (1989) published a scathing review of Department of Health and Social Security funded research (indicating the presumed quality of the grant-holders) conducted between 1975 and 1986.

None of the preceding material means that the nursing profession is unaware that it has responsibilities for research. In 1995, the English National Board for Nursing, Midwifery and Health Visiting published a report on a survey it had carried out in order to identify priorities for research in the different nursing specialities, including mental health. Its findings illustrate many of the difficulties that I discuss in this chapter, and they need to be considered carefully. The report categorises a welter of data, and ranks them into priorities that are inferred from the numbers of people who identify topics.

The appearance of one first-priority topic (the role of the nurse teacher in the clinical area) in more than one category perhaps reflects a guilty anxiety about nursing, and the report lists a number of topics that are simply uninvestigable. For example, 'an evaluation of Project 2000 learners in their first year after qualifying' demands a control group of non-Project 2000 learners, which no longer exists. The time to have done this study was when there were a number of different schemes of training running concurrently. (Naively I, with some colleagues at Kings College, London, tried to get resources for just such a project when it should have been clear to us that no one would fund a study whose findings would be published just as the implementation of Project 2000 across the country was completed.)

Other topics are uninvestigable because they will be decided by policy-makers. For example, 'boundaries of care between health and social services' will probably be changed by whichever political party wins the British general election. Other topics rest on assumptions that are themselves untested. For example, 'the implementation of clinical supervision in all areas of nursing and the outcome on patient care and professional development' assumes that clinical supervision is a unitary phenomenon and that its outcomes in different settings (themselves assumed to be unitary phenomena) are comparable. But what is most striking in the list of first priorities for research in nursing is that out of 84 topics (which include three or four duplicates), fewer than a quarter (see Crow & Stedman, 1995) refer to more or less specific interventions that might be tested as part of an evaluation of nursing care.

The report also lists the 17 highest priorities for mental health nursing, eight of which represent potentially testable interventions (one of which, the care programme approach, has already been reviewed by the Cochrane Collaboration, which regards it as in no need of further research). It also provides a non-prioritised list of mental health nursing topics (125 including numerous duplicate and overlapping items) of which fewer than half refer to potentially testable interventions.

Educational structures and nursing

It is not surprising, then, that psychiatric nurses have been peripheral to major decisions on health care taken since the general election of 1987 (Brown, 1992). The most worrying consequence of this lack of influence moves round a self-amplifying loop back to nurse education. The reorganisation of National Health Service management, the internal market, and the formation of NHS Trusts, were unanticipated by the planners of Project

2000 and of PREPP (as it was first known). But Conservative governments between 1979 and 1997 disarticulated education, as well as health care.

The School Curriculum and Assessment Authority (SCAA) and the National Council for Vocational Qualifications (NCVQ) regulate standards of the bodies that award A levels, general national vocational qualifications (GNVQs), and national vocational qualifications (NVQs). Such has been the pace of change and development that Sir Ronald Dearing was commissioned to report in 1996 on educational qualifications for 16–18 year olds, trying to respond to the perplexity of employers comparing, for example, an advanced GNVQ in science and an A level in science. He argues that students must be able to build a portfolio of qualifications across vocational and academic pathways, and that the GNVQ should be strengthened both as an alternative to A levels and a basis for the NVQ.

Not only have these organisations and qualifications developed independently of the bodies that regulate specialist education for nurses, but two of the most striking aspects of the GNVQ and NVQ programmes are the specificity and measurability of their outcomes. Because employers need be in no doubt about the key skills of someone with a level 5 GNVQ, there is little to stop them taking him or her on instead of a grade D or E registered nurse.

A central issue for nurse education will be how we map our qualifications onto other vocational and academic awards. It may become painfully clear that health providers do not need philosophers, but they do need clinicians whose demonstrable competence in their work can be observed by third parties (JICC & Mental Health Foundation, 1996, Sainsbury Centre, 1997). Dearing (1996, p. 77) says, 'A qualification like the National Vocational Qualification should not be granted unless a candidate has demonstrated all the competences necessary to provide a reliable service to a client'. In other words, 'every detailed aspect of what is involved in mastery [of a subject, trade or profession] has to be demonstrated by the candidate, and assessed' (Dearing, 1996, p. 75). The candidate repeatedly demonstrates to the assessor mastery of what is required. Of course, a key element of nursing is the discretion that individual practitioners have over their work. But how can we be assured that a nurse is competent to exercise that discretion, if we also know that much of nursing care is 'recipe knowledge' used every day, and almost entirely untested by psychiatric nurses? In what sense is the holder of an ENB 998 course formally qualified in the assessment and verification of nursing competences?

Ineffective strategies

A rough distinction between prediction and knowledge is that a prediction is an opinion, the evidence for which has not been tested, and knowledge is either an opinion for which all the relevant evidence has been tested or an opinion, the evidence for which we do not care to test. Either nursing knowledge, comprising rules for practice, is so strong that it supplants the need for written rules, or it is so common-sensical that all nurses can take it for granted (practical reasoning). However, nursing is a technology which applies scientific knowledge to skilled behaviours (see Wolpert, 1992). Unlike medicine, which is also a system where knowledge is applied to skilled behaviours, nursing has been slow to acquire scientific rationales for the services that it offers to patients. I suggested earlier that for many years, nurse education has encouraged a sense of personal authority in psychiatric nursing in order to foster a sense of moral justification for individuals' practice. This subjective sense of personal authority necessitates challenging what is seen as the dominant discipline in the mental health services and its perceived values.

If psychiatry reflects rather than shapes social structures, or if nurse education, for all its rhetoric, is simply a system for perpetuating the existing distribution of power and responsibility in the mental health services (and the rhetoric is psychiatric nurses' apologia for their participation in this traditionally class- and gender-based structure), it follows that if psychiatric care is dehumanising it is not good enough to attribute the causes to factors other than the lack of consensus among psychiatric nurses about the formulation of nursing care. Psychiatric nurses complain of the mystification of mental illness by biological psychiatrists but have not adequately addressed the possibility that biological explanations of psychiatric phenomena may be the most parsimonious, avoiding the elaborations involved in social/environmental explanations. Eliot Freidson (1975) noted that mental illness was attractive to sociologists because of the causal factors apparently definable in psychosocial terms. Sociologists saw the practice of psychiatrists as being somehow different from that of oncologists or surgeons. Aetiology of mental illness, unlike the causes of cancer, was treated 'as an imputation rather than as a fact' (Freidson, 1975, p. 225). Psychiatric nurses do not seem to have caught up with the fact that, as psychiatry and psychology have increased their ability to explain symptoms and illness behaviour, so the output of sociological work on the aetiology of mental illness has declined.

A new clerisy

Libertarian and authoritarian approaches to psychiatry are conflated, not least with respect to the issues of insight and diagnosis. Ian Kennedy (1981), like many psychiatric nurses, argues that psychiatric diagnosis is inherently wicked because it enables the psychiatrist to take control of other people by attempting to control the hypothesised illness. That is, the diagnosis disembodies the illness from the person, objectifying it and so the treatment. But consider a diagnosis of stage IV breast cancer in a woman who is the wrong side of 70. Her age enables the doctor to relinquish control of the illness, to justify not treating her because her age makes prolonging her survival a less urgent matter than prolonging the survival of a younger woman even though by now she is an 'expert' (albeit a lay expert) on her illness. Or, suppose that a man presents with symptoms of low mood, tiredness and dyspepsia that are diagnosed by his general practitioner as depression. The GP's diagnosis of depression fails to legit-imise the man's account of his illness, not because of the ascription of mental illness, but because it prevents his access to treatment for the gastric cancer that underlies his fatigue and low spirits.

In both cases the doctors fail to take the opportunity for control affor-ded by diagnosis, thus preventing the patients from taking part in the phase that follows diagnosis – negotiation and choice of treatment. Heath (1992) has observed that in British general practice patients receive diagnostic information quite passively. Schizophrenia and bipolar dis-order are no different from cancer, in that the reception of diagnostic information is likely to be culturally influenced (for example by class and education) rather than an effect of the diagnostic process itself. Diagnosis therefore does not preclude attempts to mediate between self and illness. By denying the legitimacy of diagnosis nurses run the risk of colluding in the false belief that in being diagnosed as having cancer, schizo-phrenia or bipolar disorder, one's self is somehow invalidated and, worse, one's ability to negotiate and choose one's treatment is also invali-dated. Diagnosis (and disagreement about diagnosis) might rather be a key area where a mutually interdependent attempt is made to mediate between the internal reality of the patient and the external world in which the patient is obliged to make his or her way. Diagnosis becomes then not a fixed point of resolution but a starting point for learning how to balance opposing tensions.

Empiricism and strongly held world-views are not incompatible, for a person has to declare his or her world-view in order for an observer to evaluate that person's declarations. The fact that nursing knowledge is based in part on science does not mean that nurses are necessarily scien-tists. Nurses are in a good position to observe science, bringing to bear a moral perspective informed by the other disciplines on which nursing is based. But if their observation of science remains from the viewpoint of the outsider then how can they mediate between patients and psy-chiatry? And how can they argue that their viewpoint is any more valu-able than those of the general public and its elected representatives? If nurses take it upon themselves to be the moral arbiters of how scientific knowledge is to be applied in psychiatry then they place themselves above critical debate of their own role in a democracy. It has been argued that so-called qualitative research is based on different defini-tions of evidence, reason, logic, observation, perception, confirmation and probability.

However, Eco *et al.* (1992) rebut such a view, showing that interpretation of empirical observations (however gathered and recorded) is the basis of all theory, including literary theory. Can it possibly be ethical to practise on other human beings on the basis of undeclared faith whose tenets are not available for another observer to interpret and evaluate? I suggest that ironic reflexivity, entailed by a social constructivist view, might be suitable for certain kinds of academic debate, but is likely only to perplex a psy-chotic recipient of a psychiatric nurse's services.

Independence of service users

Many of the National Health Service reforms of the 1980s and 1990s were aimed at removing from health care professionals their power as purchasing agents on behalf of patients. This means that the purchasing agent is now a bureaucracy rather than an individual professional, and it is certainly not the patient acting as his or her own agent. It is possible to set standards for services in the absence of substantive nursing knowledge but can they be justified to individual users of services and their carers and families? Psychiatric nurses who too readily adopt new ideas, and nurses who fail to keep up with current developments in psychology and medicine, are not necessarily so different from each other.

The Cochrane Collaboration's (Cochrane Library, 1996) systematic evaluation of clinical effectiveness is important not only for nurses but also for service users who, perhaps for the first time, have access to information on a range of mental health interventions. The Cochrane database greatly enhances their ability to make an informed choice about their treatment. One of its systematic reviews incidentally also suggests what service user groups have argued for some time; that what is valuable about case management is not the management of the case, but assertive community outreach that builds on users' strengths rather than (as Peter Campbell, a founder-member of Survivors Speak Out, has scornfully said) educating them out of their mad ideas.

The words 'mediation', 'medicine', 'remedy' and 'median' may all have a similar origin. The word 'broker' (sometimes used instead of 'mediator') undoubtedly originates from mercantile practice. It seems suitable that 'broker' entered the nursing lexicon during the reorganisation of the health services in the United Kingdom in the 1990s. A genuinely user-led agenda requires nurses to accept that they, along with other health care providers, are part of a dominant social structure that can be changed only by political action that places service users in key planning positions, and that targets most resources to areas of greatest need (Thornicroft & Strathdee, 1996).

Enforcing versus enabling

Psychiatric nursing care can be conceptualised on a number of dimensions, including that of enforcing/enabling. Despite most nurses' rejection of a so-called medical model, psychiatric nurses, attempting to maximise the ambiguities of their work, become enforcers rather than enablers. I am currently collaborating with the nurses and other staff on a number of projects in a unit that practises non-biological psychiatry. That is not to say that it eschews biologically-based interventions but that these interventions are part of a range on offer to the clients of the service, most of whom are highly critical of the unit even while they develop attachments to its staff. In this I suspect they are not unlike William Styron who regarded most of the staff during his hospital admission for depression with sceptical warmth, deriding them for their naive assumption that their interventions contributed to his recovery. Styron's attitude to the psychiatric staff does not obscure his view of his depression from which he draws two conclusions. One (which can be contrasted with Ian Kennedy's 1981 view) is that had he killed himself, as he probably would have done if he had not been admitted to hospital, it would not have been a rational and free exercise of choice and responsibility for himself, but a 'simulacrum of all the evil of our world' (Styron, 1991, p. 83). The second is that 'the genetic roots of depression seem now to be beyond controversy' (Styron, 1991, p. 79).

We need to attend to Styron's derision. Firstly, he does not even bother to mention the nursing staff. Secondly, he regards the psychological therapies on offer as infantile, or condescending and bullying. What contributed most to his recovery, despite an undoubtedly biologically and partially genetically determined disorder, were seclusion (not a banged-up-in-solitary type of seclusion) and time within a place that, while it was a madhouse, was less of a madhouse than his home had become. Styron's observation recalls a suggestion by Peter Campbell that a core competence for a psychiatric nurse should be the ability to stay for hours at a time, if necessary, with a person in crisis in his or her own home, as opposed to the ability to keep an inpatient shut in a side room while seated outside the door reading a newspaper. An even more derisive view is expressed by H.G. Woodley (1947, p. 71): 'Not to everyone is afforded the opportunity of being a sane man in a lunatic asylum; but to all asylum nurses stands open the door through which they can contribute greatly in making the lives around them happier and better. Why they foolishly suggest punching the old bastard in the guts, I simply do not know ... '.

Vernacular versus technical competence

T.S. Eliot (1957), who experienced mental illness personally (as did his wife), suggested that problems of explanation in psychiatry were similar to problems of explanation in literary criticism. Understanding a poem and understanding 'troubled individuals' are, Eliot suggests, not only matters of investigation of components and origins or causes of the trouble, but of 'endeavouring to grasp its entelechy' (Eliot, 1957, p. 110). He says, '...the literary critic is not merely a technical expert, who has learned the rules to be observed by the writers he criticises: the critic must be the whole man, a man with convictions and principles, and knowledge and experience of life' (Eliot, 1957, p. 116).

I would like to extend Eliot's suggestion and ask whether the literary critic can contribute to an understanding of psychiatric nursing. Can convictions, principles, knowledge and experience coexist with the way that many nurses use language? But first, why does it matter? Orwell (1961, p. 353) thought it was worth worrying because incompetent language 'makes it easier for us to have foolish thoughts'. Simms' (1978) observation that the semantic organisation of the psychiatric nurse's lexicon could illuminate the ways in which nurses acquire practical knowledge is borne out by a range of studies into the way that professionals talk to and about their clients or patients (Drew & Heritage, 1992). So far from being agents of demystification, psychiatric nurses work in a vernacularly-characterised setting (as Steve Tilley, 1995, showed in his research) in which the vernacular is used 'recurrently and pervasively' (see Drew & Heritage, 1992, p. 26) to specify and maintain the norms of the institution, not necessarily located in a building.

Jargon is not just an idle evasion of a need to state precisely what has gone on between nurse and patient in a clinical setting. If a person masturbates in a crowded day room the label 'socially inappropriate behaviour' appears to avoid expression of a judgement, sounds like a neutral report and, most importantly, does not sound like a value-laden reason for enforcement of physical or psychological coercion. Another strategy is the use of pathologising language to describe someone who has no symptoms of mental disorder: for example, 'Mr Smith is not expressing any delusions', or 'No inappropriate behaviour or speech noted'. Another way in which the nurse enforces his or her view of the patient's needs or problems is to use doubt both to avoid commitment to a judgement, and to suggest that a professional assessment has taken place: for example, 'Mr Smith gives the appearance of being cheerful'. The language is entirely normative, but importantly appears non-judgemental (see Simms, 1978)

Health care records are not the only place to find jargon. Nurses (and I include myself) have always tended to fasten on to terms or ideas, such as the nursing process which caused me a great deal of grief when I first became a charge nurse. There is a sinister side to this tendency that I will explore via the word 'mentor'.

Mentor was, until discovered by nurses and management theorists, a dying metaphor derived not even directly from Homer's Odyssey but via a sanctimonious archbishop's version of the story of Telemachus (Fénelon, 1931). Its archaism is pretentiously used to give a false appearance of tradition to a new (and unevaluated) experiment in nurse education. Strictly speaking it is meaningless. No two workers agree on its meaning. The use of the term 'mentor' would matter less if there was a conscious dishonesty, but somehow the linguistic swindlers' seeming ignorance makes it worse.

Homer recounts the degradation in Telemachus' household, with suitors pestering his mother and reports that his father is missing, presumed dead. Homer adds a puzzle about who the real Mentor is. Is he the pompous and ineffectual old gentleman whom Odysseus left to take care of his affairs and who quite clearly has not done so, or is he the goddess with the flashing eyes who uses Mentor's appearance to help Telemachus find his father and to take revenge on the disloyal Ithacans? Homer's account shows that Mentor (a man) did not amount to much without the intervention of Athene (a goddess). Mentor/Athene helps to bring Telemachus to a new relationship with his father, on the way helping him to grow up, these being the themes elaborated by Fénelon (1931).

Is any of this anything remotely to do with the responsibilities of the nurse instructor in clinical settings? I have seen the term 'mentoring programme'. This suggests that there might be a verb 'to mentor', and an adjective 'mentorable', as in, 'I have been mentoring this nurse unsuccessfully for three months', or 'This nurse is quite unmentorable', or 'Despite constant mentoring this nurse's work remains unsatisfactory'. The symbolic nature of the word 'mentor' clearly implies something more than a verbal sign for a clinical instructor, but although it could be argued that communication is enhanced by the extension of symbolic meaning beyond dictionary definitions, 'mentor' peddles the connotations of philosophy and even ideology while actually concealing a fragmented and uncertain group of people who cannot agree among themselves what words like 'nursing', 'learning' and 'caring' mean when applied to practical action. What sounds like an idea is a reification of partially understood aspects of interaction between people elevated to an ideology.

As with all ideology there is a logical gulf between the rhetoric and the actions of the people who espouse it. That nurses are notoriously bad at defining, operationalising and testing the components of nursing adds to the confusion about how to acquire the skills to be a nurse, let alone a mentor. Worst of all, 'mentor' exemplifies the moral superiority that justifies one nurse meddling in the private thoughts of another, the moral superiority that is justified by critical theory, and the meddling that is justified by the nurse's privileged status as an agent of demystification. I suggest that part of a nurse's socialisation is his or her demonstration of competence in the lexicon (jargon/vernacular) of nursing, rather than competence in nursing actions and interventions. Jargon used purportedly to account for a nurse's actions actually functions to protect him or her from accountability for his or her actions.

A clinical experiment that failed

Although I think that it is possible both to hold a medicalised view of mental illness and to try to help a person to reconstitute his or her inner world while retaining his or her individual autonomy, I think there are serious risks in such an enterprise. Dewey (1963) argued that one of the purposes of education was to regard all ideas as hypotheses to be tested. New staff would come to the ward in which I worked for 6 years, expecting to be unconditionally accepted by existing staff and patients simply because they 'believed in' psychotherapy; whereas we actually believed that individual, dyadic and group reflection on the relationship between nurse and patient provided the basis for extraction of the 'net meanings which are the capital stock for intelligent dealing with future experiences' (Dewey, 1963, p. 87). Newcomers' resentment could be mortifying both for them and us when their formulation of the idea of psychotherapy was questioned, repeatedly and not always very politely.

Authenticity was not enough. We aimed to engage both staff and patients in the kind of inquiry that was driven by collective debate (always, we hoped, rational) and aimed to uncover meaning. Such inquiry entails toleration of conflict within and between its participants.

Without tolerance people could not be expected to bring into open view bitter and feared memories. But while we demanded the commitment that is entailed by validation and verification (Polanyi, 1962), an anthropologist observing the ward thought that the ward's principles of plurality and democracy were continually undermined by unresolved conflicts over identity and status.

In another, not always explicit conflict, our so-called millenarian attempt to deconstruct authority risked being undermined by our reliance on psychoanalysts to help engender meaning out of chaotic events. The charismatic authority of the analyst encouraged individuals to objectify the interpretations, as if the clash between internal and external worlds could be fixed and resolved once and for all. We always ran the twin risks of forgetting that any statement by any person could only ever be a hypothesis, and reverting to the exercise of hierarchical authority vested in a defensive bureaucracy of meetings, decisions postponed, and debate stifled in routine.

We believed that what we were doing was right and so, as Carlo Maria Giulini observed when conducting an orchestra, we worked together because of that, not because we were ordered to. The trouble was that our socio-analytical methods led to results that were impossible to replicate. It may be that we lacked the technology required to accomplish the changes in nursing care that we wished, but perhaps the technology was available and we as a group were still unable to synchronise our efforts enough to take advantage of it. A fixed and rigid ward organisation is easier to monitor than one that is continuously changing. A simple, undifferentiated system of nursing care is easier to administer than the differentiated, multi-system organisation of primary nursing.

We tried to make our interventions multi-purpose rather than anchored to specific tasks. We tried to organise ourselves participatively and democratically rather than autocratically and paternalistically. We expected all members of the ward (patients and staff) to be social rather than isolated. And our data were non-verifiable; partly because of gross shortcomings in record-keeping (records often lacked dates, or signatures by nurses, or page numbers, or patients' names on individual charts and record sheets); partly because of the discretion exercised by primary nurses; and partly because many decisions arose from conflict, interaction, and the constantly changing environment.

Perhaps our reliance on group dynamics and psychodynamics obscured our view of societal influences like racism (we treated very few Black patients), class (we treated many middle-class and professional patients), and sexism (we were slow to recognise the disproportionate number of women who had experienced sexual assault as children). We had attempted to apply what Sue Pembrey (1980) had concluded from her research into the role of the ward sister – that individualised nursing care could only occur when the charge nurse systematically retrieved accountability reports from nurses on the discretion they exercised over their work, and met all patients face-to-face and every day. In attempting to practise holistic nursing we thought we could improve individuals' mental health without taking too much notice of the social processes that generate illness and disability, nor of the social processes of a psychiatric hospital (see Williams, 1993).

I have found to my cost that although, for instance, people with anorexia are members of a particular kind of society whose demands exert a pathoplastic effect on the expression of the disorder, trying to engage a starving young women in a discussion of her role as victim of society (and what is this but a pat diagnosis?) may have lethal consequences if it is used as the main intervention in her anorexia. Violent behaviour, so greatly feared in schizophrenia, no less by nurses than the general public, seems to be one way of trying to regain control from the passivity symptoms that are such a demoralising feature of the disorder. But to refrain from intervening in violent behaviour simply because its meaning can be understood may lead to great harm, again as I have found to my cost.

The relationship of biological responses to experience of psychological trauma is far from clear, but 'nervous shock' is recognised in law (and by the people who experience it) as both profoundly disabling and stigmatising. Like people with post-traumatic stress disorder, people with schizophrenia and anorexia are no less moral and social agents, and are likely to refuse treatment, but that does not support an argument for denying the existence of the disorders, nor for regarding them as purely socially constructed phenomena. We often lost sight of the fact that the main purpose of interpreting our observations was to decide whether we were offering the right kind of care, not to search for meaning as an end in itself.

Ambiguity and victimhood in the therapeutic relationship

Passivity symptoms do not make a person with schizophrenia a passive recipient of nursing care. Lack of knowledge about the causes and natural history of schizophrenia does not invalidate attempts to ameliorate its effects, any more than lack of knowledge about the causes and natural history of psoriasis invalidates attempts to ameliorate *its* effects. As it happens, the nursing literature on both disorders is equally lacking in hard evidence for clinical practice. By ascribing victimhood to psychiatric patients nurses can feel comfortable with their power and ignore their own personal responsibility as moral agents. Indeed it is a short step to regarding oneself also as a victim of the power relations of the mental health services. In the regional conferences conducted during and after the review of mental health nursing in England (HMSO, 1994) the theme of psychiatric nurses as victims was constant. Service users repeatedly observed that while nurses felt victimised they were likely to victimise patients. I suggest that the ascription of victim status to self as well as to patient may be made by a nurse who nonetheless continues to perceive him or herself as a moral agent. This places patients at risk.

'I am abused and I abuse
I am the victim and I am the perpetrator
I am innocent and I am innocent
I am guilty and I am guilty'

(Rose 1992, p. 294)

Rose's 'dialectical lyric' satirises the paradox that Michael Moorcock (1995) identifies: if you want to know where free speech ends and corruption begins, don't ask a pornographer. Mental illness and sex both undermine political power. Mental illness and sex both undermine society's control over money and other property. Just as pornography exploits and corrupts for profit the power imbalance that is always latent in our most intimate relationships, so therapy risks exploiting and corrupting for profit the power imbalance between the helper and the helped who necessarily exposes his or her needs to scrutiny (measurement) with no guarantee that they will be met. Moorcock suggests that society's confusion about pornography prevents it from holding commercial enterprises accountable for the effects of their actions in publishing material depicting the brutalisation of children and women. Is it likely that commercial enterprises (for such are universities and hospitals now) will be held accountable for the effects of their failures to produce (!) safe and effective practitioners of the healing arts?

Complicity in the new economic order for the health services

Psychiatric nurses have acquiesced in the introduction of managed competition which has brought with it an increase in the numbers of support workers, and a gender-determined social structure for health care workers generally. The larger proportion of support workers are women, ultimately managed by men, although nominally under the control of other women (e.g. staff nurses). The alliance of senior women in nursing with the senior men whose numbers predominate is also an alliance with the existing order of gender-relations and economic distribution. Men are disproportionately represented in senior posts (by definition now general managers), and also among those entering psychiatric nursing with first degrees. If the best educated people lead the profession where does that leave the most skilled, and how does the profession deal with this issue? If the most skilled people lead the profession where does that leave the best educated, and how does the profession deal with this issue?

I suggest that these are questions that ought to make us extremely sceptical of attacks led by men on the men of other professions, for what better smoke screen for the marginalisation of women in nursing? Dearing's (1996) suggestion (expressed though it is in gender-specific language) that a key aim of the system of national vocational qualifications is to eliminate gender bias has a bearing on the status of women in the health care professions generally and, inevitably, on the status of women in psychiatric nursing. The better education of the few under Project 2000 is being accomplished in a way that both exploits and augments the material and political poverty of the disadvantaged, partly represented by the women who provide low or unwaged and non-technical care, partly by the patients who hitherto have not had access to the information to enable them to choose between methods of care. I suggest that it is no bad thing if this is challenged by the system of general national vocational qualifications.

The purpose of mediation

Mediation is the management of ambiguity. A major purpose of mediation is, in David Selbourne's (1994, p. 164) words, 'the restoration to the estranged individual, and to the civic order to which he ostensibly belongs, of his social being'. I have suggested that nurses reject what they perceive to be the civic order while they behave in ways that actually strengthen existing social structures. The common law, the law of tort and related judicial decisions have probably had greater influence on nursing practice than arguments about what nurses do or don't know.

The common law and legislation both depend on interpretation by 'reasonable' practitioners of law and nursing. Three problems ensue. Firstly, the process depends on the existence of reasonable practitioners, whether of the law or of nursing. Secondly, if the practice of nursing is shaped by forces that are essentially outside the control of nurses, then the potential for ambiguity and its exploitation for personal gain are maximised, despite the apparent threat of legal sanctions. Thirdly, there is a problem with the concept of 'reasonableness' itself. Selbourne (1994, p. 68) argues that adherence to a notion of 'reasonableness' has led, in part, to a false belief that 'morally benign purposes will generally prevail in the civic order over malign intentions'. I have tried to show that psychiatric nurses' moral justification of their practice has contributed to harm to patients.

Accounting for practice

In being unable to justify their practice with the kind of evidence offered by a randomised controlled trial of a treatment/intervention, or by longitudinal studies or by single-case studies, nurses are also unable to justify (account for) why they rather than anyone else should mediate between the internal worlds of estranged individuals and the outside worlds of which they are necessarily a part. Evidence-based practice is an account that can be morally justified because it is rational (not in the scientific sense but in the sense with which I began this chapter). It is a system of practice whose beliefs and goals cohere with its actions and so the Cochrane Collaboration is able to delimit debate about medical treatments.

Settling the issue of which is the most effective treatment does not settle the political and social consequences of closing the argument. For example, it may be that the most effective pharmaceutical treatment for a common illness is the most costly, or that an uncommon but high-profile illness can be effectively treated by a cheap-to-manufacture but patented drug. These outcomes have implications for politicians. A likely outcome in psychiatry is that the most effective treatments are combinations of physiological and psychosocial interventions, the balance of which depends on the characteristics of the individual patient. This outcome entails not only challenging politicians to fund the integrated and comprehensive services required to assess need for and to deliver these combined interventions, but also challenging the vested interests of the professional groups comprising mental health and social services.

It is at this point that critical theories, especially those associated with the Frankfurt school (Geuss, 1981), can contribute to explanations of how and why social institutions act as they do. It is also indisputably helpful to understand the nature of discourse and its relationship to praxis (bearing in mind that Foucault's (1972) is not the only account of discourse). Analysis of the social settings of psychiatric nurses' work with patients may occur in a range of dimensions – functional, structural, lexical – but each analytical dimension implies similar constraints on the analysts. These constraints can be described from the perspectives of 'stranger' and 'native'. To say that there is more to nursing than the interventions nurses carry out in their work with patients, is not to say that nurses (natives) are in the best position to try to identify and correct the profession's perceptual biases. On the other hand, to adapt Warnock's (1957) analysis, nurses may simply be looking in the wrong direction when they look to philosophy and sociology to answer questions about their day-to-day practice. Nor because nurses look to them are philosophers and sociologists (strangers) obliged to give answers about day-to-day practice.

The lack of evidence for establishing the minimum 'nursing' course units needed for an academic award in nursing that also comes with a statutory qualification means that research into nursing interventions and actions is urgently needed. For example, nurses need to grasp the basis of professional ethics, but they do not need to be philosophers. Solving the problem of vernacular versus technical competence is central to educating nurses to take their places as equals of the other professions in the mental health services. If 3-year education programmes for nurses are to stay, I predict that they will be found to be too short to allow elective courses that are not focused on the competencies of psychiatric nursing, practised under full supervision, and assessed by properly qualified assessors.

In the current circumstances, at worst, a few qualified nurses (CPNs, health visitors, district nurses) are employed to prevent ill-health (i.e. contamination of the better-off by the poor and diseased) and to educate (i.e. police the individual's lifestyle), while the real abuses of our society (the acquisition of power by economic exploitation or physical violence or both) go unchecked – the poor, diseased, and ineducable winding up in run-for-profit institutions, including prisons. At best, as the Royal College of Nursing Institute and the Royal College of Psychiatrists (Ward, 1996) are showing, psychiatric nurses are front-line providers in a network of community mental health teams which have solved the problems of separate social and mental health services budgets, which try to enable patients to live productive lives in spite of their severe mental illnesses, and which might be approaching what Peter Sedgwick described as a cross-sectional alliance in an ethical structure of fellowship and solidarity. But I very much doubt whether more than a handful of university nursing departments conduct research projects or run courses that are directly relevant to this work.

References

Ayllon, T. & Azrin, N.H. (1964) Reinforcement and instructions with mental patients. *Journal of the Experimental Analysis of Behaviour* 7, 327–331.

Ayllon, T. & Haughton, E. (1964) Modification of symptomatic verbal behaviour of mental patients. *Behaviour Research & Therapy* 2, 87–97.

Brown, J. (1992) European legislation and mental health nursing. Paper delivered to the Mental Health Nursing Conference held at the University of East Anglia, Norwich, 18–19 September, 1992.

The Cochrane Library (1996) *Cochrane Collaboration, Issue 3*. Update Software, Oxford.

Crow, S. & Stedman, S. (1995) *Report of the National Consultation to Identify Research Priorities in Nursing Midwifery and Health Visiting Education and Practice*. ENB, London.

Dearing, R. (1996) *Review of Qualifications for 16–19 Year Olds*. School Curriculum and Assessment Authority, Hayes.

Dewey, J. (1963) *Experience of Education*. Collier Macmillan, London.

Drew, P. & Heritage, J. (1992) Analyzing talk at work. In *Talk at Work* (P. Drew & J. Heritage eds), Cambridge University Press, Cambridge.

Eco, U., Rorty, R., Culler, J., Brooke-Rose, C. & Collini, S. (1992) *Interpretation and Over-interpretation*. Cambridge University Press, Cambridge.

Eliot, T.S. (1957) *On Poetry and Poets*. Faber, London.

Evans, M. (1995) The use of knowledge in nursing and psychotherapy as a defence against unbearable experiences. Paper presented at the Association of Psychoanalytic Psychotherapy in the NHS Inaugural Nursing SubCommittee Conference, 28 October 1995. Tavistock, London.

Fénelon, F. de S. de la M. (1931) (1717) *Extraits: Aventures de Télemaque, Fables, Dialogues des Morts* (A. Cahen & P. Richardot eds). Librairie Hachette, Paris.

Foucault, M. (1972) *The Archaeology of Knowledge*. Tavistock, London.

Freidson, E. (1975) *Profession of Medicine*. Dodd Mead & Co., New York.

Geuss, R. (1981) *The Idea of a Critical Theory*. Cambridge University Press, Cambridge.

Guttenplan, S. (1994) *A Companion to the Philosophy of Mind*. Basil Blackwell, Oxford.

Heath, C. (1992) Diagnosis in the general practice consultation. In *Talk at Work* (P. Drew & J. Heritage eds). Cambridge University Press, Cambridge.

HMSO (1994) *Working in Partnership*. HMSO, London.

Joint Initiative for Community Care/Mental Health Foundation (1996) *Study into the Qualifications and Training for Care Staff and Volunteers Working with Adults of Pre-retirement Age who are Mentally Ill in Residential and Non-residential Services in the Statutory and Independent Sectors*. JICC, Milton Keynes.

Kennedy, I. (1981) *The Unmasking of Medicine*. George Allen & Unwin, London.

Littlewood, J. (1991) Care and ambiguity: towards a concept of nursing. In *Anthropology in Nursing* (P. Holden & J. Littlewood eds). Routledge, London.

Moorcock, M. (1995) *Demons, Delight and Erotic Instincts. Uncensored, Part 3.* The Observer, London.

Orwell, G. (1961) *Collected Essays.* Secker & Warburg, London.

Pembrey, S. (1980) *The Ward Sister: Key to Nursing.* Royal College of Nursing, London.

Polanyi, M. (1962) *Personal Knowledge.* Routledge & Kegan Paul, London.

Ritter, S. (1989) *Bethlem Royal and Maudsley Hospitals Manual of Clinical Psychiatric Nursing Principles and Procedures.* Harper and Row, London.

Robinson, J. & Elkan, R. (1989) *Research for Policy and Policy for Research: A Review of Selected DHSS-Funded Nurse Education Research 1975–1986.* Nursing Policy Studies Centre, University of Warwick, Warwick.

Rose, G. (1992) *The Broken Middle.* Blackwell Science, Oxford.

Sainsbury Centre (1997) *Review of the Rules and Training of Mental Health Care Staff: Report of the Working Group.* Sainsbury Centre for Mental Health, London.

Sedgwick, P. (1982) *Psychopolitics.* Pluto, London.

Selbourne, D. (1994) *The Principle of Duty.* Sinclair-Stevenson, London.

Sills, G.M. (1977) Research in the field of psychiatric nursing. *Nursing Research* **26** (3), 122–128.

Simms, J.A. (1978) The social organization of psychiatric nursing: theoretical comments upon sociological and hospital research and empirical observation of the behaviour of nursing staff. PhD thesis, University of Manchester Department of Management Sciences, Manchester.

Steering Group (1996) *Report of the Confidential Enquiry into Homicides and Suicides by Mentally Ill People.* Royal College of Psychiatry, London.

Styron, W. (1991) *Darkness Visible.* Jonathan Cape, London.

Thornicroft, G. & Strathdee, G. (1996) *Commissioning Mental Health Services.* HMSO, London.

Tilley, S. (1995) *Negotiating Realities.* Avebury, Aldershot.

Ward, M. (1996) Interim report on survey of caseloads and management skills in community mental health teams. Paper delivered at the National Institute for Nursing Conference, St Catherine's College, Oxford, 5 November 1996.

Warnock, G.J. (1957) Analysis and imagination. In *Revolution in Philosophy* (A.J. Ayer *et al.* eds). Macmillan, London.

Williams, W.P. (1993) *Aspects of a therapeutic milieu.* PhD thesis, University College, London.

Wolpert, L. (1992) *The Unnatural Nature of Science.* Faber and Faber, London.

Woodley, H.G. (1947) *Certified: An Autobiographical Study.* Gollancz, London.

Wynne, L.C. (1978) Knotted relationships. In *Beyond the Double Bind* (M.M. Berger ed.). Brunner Mazel, New York.

Further reading

Abbondanza, D., Puskar, K.R., Wilkinson, B., Welch, C., Rudert, S. & Gallippi, B. (1994) Psychiatric mental health nursing in a biopsychosocial era. *Perspectives in Psychiatric Care* **30** (3), 21–25.

Allport, G.W. (1938) *Personality: A Psychological Interpretation.* Constable, London.

Auerswald, E.H. (1968) Interdisciplinary versus ecological approach. *Family Process* **7**, 202–215.

Barker, P., Baldwin, S. & Ulas, M. (1989) Medical expansionism. *Nurse Education Today* **9**, 192–202.

Barker, P., Reynolds, B. & Ward, T. (1995) The proper focus of nursing: a critique of the 'caring' ideology. *International Journal of Nursing Studies* **32** (4), 386–397.

Baruch, G. & Treacher, A. (1978) *Psychiatry Observed*. Routledge & Kegan Paul, London.
The Rule of St Benedict for Monasteries (1969) translated by Dom BB Bolton.
Berger, M.M. (1978) *Beyond the Double Bind*. Brunner Mazel, New York.
Bernard, C. (1957) *An Introduction to the Study of Experimental Medicine*. Constable, London.
Blankesteijn, H. & Hacquebrod, L. (1993) God and the Arctic survivors. *New Scientist* **138** (1867), 38–42.
Boreham, N.C. (1978) Test skill interaction errors in the assessment of nurses' clinical proficiency. *Journal of Occupational Psychology* **51**, 249–258.
Boswell, J. (1988) *The Kindness of Strangers*. Penguin, Harmondsworth.
Brody, E.B. (1982) Are we for mental health as well as against mental illness? *American Journal of Psychiatry* **139**, 1588–1589.
Brunswik, E. (1952) *The Conceptual Framework of Psychology*. University of Chicago Press, Chicago.
Burrell, G. (1989) *Buster's Fired a Wobbler*. Penguin, Harmondsworth.
Coulter, J. (1973) *Approaches to Insanity*. Martin Robertson, London.
Culyer, A.J. (1994) *Supporting Research & Development in the National Health Service: Report of the Research & Development Task Force*. HMSO, London.
Dillon, G.L. (1991) *Contending Rhetorics*. Indiana University Press, Bloomington.
Drew, B.J. (1988) Devaluation of biological knowledge. *IMAGE Journal of Nursing Scholarship* **20** (1), 25–26.
Eagleton, T. (1991) *Ideology*. Verso, London.
Farr, R.M. (1978) On the varieties of social psychology: an essay on the relationship between psychology and other social sciences. *Social Science Information* **17** (4–5), 503–525.
Goldberg, D. & Huxley, P. (1992) *Common Mental Disorders*. Routledge, London.
Handy, J. (1990) *Occupational Stress in a Caring Profession: the Social Context*. Avebury, Aldershot.
HMSO (1992) *The Case of Gary Harrington: Committee of Inquiry into Complaints about Ashworth Hospital Volume II*. HMSO, London.
HMSO (1994) *Working Partnership*. HMSO, London.
Horwitz, A. (1979) Models, muddles and mental illness labelling. *Journal of Health and Social Behaviour* **20**, 296–308.
Hume, D. (1966) *Enquiries Concerning the Human Understanding and Concerning the Principles of Morals*. Oxford University Press, Oxford.
Huxley, P., Hughes, J. & Challis, D. (1996) *Effective Partnerships in Mental Health: A Review of the Literature*. PSSRU, MHSWRU, University of Manchester, Manchester.
Ingleby, D. (1981) *Critical Psychiatry*. Penguin, Harmondsworth.
Jackson, M. & Williams, P. (1994) *Unimaginable Storms*. Karnac, London.
Jaspers, K. (1968) The phenomenological approach in psychopathology. *British Journal of Psychiatry* **114**, 1313–1323.
Joint Initiative for Community Care/Mental Health Foundation (1996) *Study into the Qualifications and Training for Care Staff and Volunteers Working with Adults of Pre-Retirement Age who are Mentally Ill in Residential and Non-Residential Services in the Statutory and Independent Sectors*. JICC, Milton Keynes.
Kaplan, B. (1964) *The Inner World of Mental Illness*. Harper and Row, New York.
Kernberg, O. (1980) *Internal World External Reality*. Aronson, New York.
Lamb, H.R. (1982) *Treating the Longterm Mentally Ill*. Jossey-Bass, San Francisco.
Lowery, B.J. (1993) Response to 'The common sense model: an organising framework for knowledge development in nursing'. *Scholarly Inquiry for Nursing Practice: An International Journal* **7** (2), 91–94.

Matthews, J.R. (1995) *Quantification and the Quest for Medical Certainty.* Princeton University Press, Princeton, New Jersey.

Medvedev, Z.A. & Medvedev, R.A. (1974) *The Question of Madness.* Penguin, Harmondsworth.

Moustakas, C. (1994) *Phenomenological Research Methods.* Sage, Thousand Oaks, California.

Olson, T. (1996) Fundamental and special: the dilemma of psychiatric-mental health nursing. *Archives of Psychiatric Nursing* **10** (1), 3–10.

Porter, S. (1993) Nursing research conventions: objectivity of obfuscation? *Journal of Advanced Nursing* **18**, 137–143.

Porter, S. (1993) The determinants of psychiatric nursing practice: a comparison of sociological perspectives. *Journal of Advanced Nursing* **18**, 1559–1566.

Rich, M. (1995) The bomb that didn't go off. *Financial Times*, 17 February, 1995.

Rosen, G. (1968) *Madness in Society: Chapters in the Historical Sociology of Mental Illness.* University of Chicago Press, Chicago.

Ryan, D. (1992) *Ambiguity in nursing: the patient and the ward as contrasting sources of meaning in nursing practice.* Discussion paper, The University of Edinburgh.

Sargant, W. (1971) *The Unquiet Mind.* Pan, London.

Sipe, R.B. (1983) Reification in everyday life: a psychosocial model for radical therapy. *Issues in Radical Therapy* **11** (3), 20–25, 48–56.

Smart, C. (1972) *The Religious Poetry* (M. Walsh ed.). Fyfield Books, Oxford.

Stone, D.H. (1987) A method of deriving definitions of specific competencies. *Medical Teacher* **9** (2), 155–159.

Sullivan, H.S. (1953) *The Interpersonal Theory of Psychiatry.* W.W. Norton, New York.

Swartz, M., Caroll, D. & Blazer, D.G. (1989) Psychiatric diagnosis as reified measurement. *Journal of Health and Social Behaviour* **30** (1), 33–34.

Tennyson, A. (1969) (1880) *In the Children's Hospital.* In *The Poems of Tennyson* (C. Ricks ed.). Longmans, Green & Co.

Tomlinson, B. (1992) *Report of the Inquiry into London's Health Service, Medical Education and Research.* HMSO, London.

Ward, E. (1993) The common sense model: an organising framework for knowledge development in nursing. *Scholarly Inquiry for Nursing Practice: An International Journal* **7** (2), 79–90.

Watts, A.W. (1951) *The Wisdom of Insecurity.* Vintage Books, New York.

8   Ambiguity in Nursing: The Person and the Organisation as Contrasting Sources of Meaning in Nursing

Desmond Ryan

'It is a peculiarity of occupational activities that many of the problems they pose are preset by social-institutional objectives and technological conditions. But even preset problems may be subjectively reconstituted.'

(Scribner, 1986, p. 21)

I have come to see the hospital nurse[1] as an ambiguous figure. The term 'ambiguous' I use in its accepted sense, as suggesting that the term 'nurse' can be understood in two ways. I say ambiguous 'figure' to emphasise that I am not saying that nursing attracts ambiguous types of people. Rather I see the ambiguity of the hospital nurse as a property of its being a role located in the hospital ward, much as the 'ambiguity' of amphibians (frogs, newts, etc.) expresses the dual character of the pond-plus-environs they have as their ecological niche. If the nurse is a species of human amphibian, it is because he or she inhabits simultaneously two different worlds: the world of artificial organisations and the world of natural persons. Living a double life in a dual world requires considerable versatility. This paper tries to support nurses' efforts to develop that versatility by analysing the forces for fragmentation which may prevail in the organisational environment.[2]

While I shall end by emphasising how this ambiguity, if accepted actively as a tension rather than experienced passively as a split, is the source of much of the richness which makes nursing challenging, I start from my observation that their ambiguity is not well understood by many nurses, and consequently not always well managed. I have also observed that, where it is not well managed, suffering results, not least for nurses themselves. Because it is hard to manage something which you cannot actually see, the main aim of the paper is to try to make explicit, as an aid to their better management, the situational dynamics from which derive both the ambiguity and the suffering. What follows is therefore both analytical and prescriptive, an ambiguity appropriate to the paper's human subject. Though not, of course, to the conventions of academic papers – a contradiction which will be looked into.

Ambiguity: Personhood and the Hospital Ward

'The meaning,' we used to intone, 'is the use' (Wittgenstein, 1953, p. 1).

Like words, things mean in context. Contexts are socially defined. Meaning is thus a collective project, so situations where people are collectively organized are privileged sites for meaning-giving. As well as their output of goods and services, therefore, organisations 'produce' the people who work in them (Schumacher, 1979, p. 73). Therefore we must look to the hospital ward, as a people-productive environment, for the meaning of the nurse. How should we see this environment? What is a ward?

Let's begin by following the hints from ordinary language. When nurses 'go on' a ward they 'join the ward team', much as when sailors go 'on board' a new ship they 'join' the ship's crew. This familiar terminology gives us a whole/parts situation: the ward is the whole, the ship; the ward staff are the parts, the crew. We know that hospitals and ships are not single-handed enterprises, so this language does not surprise us. We should perhaps be disquieted if similar terminology be used of the experience of patients when they come into the ward. Let me remember a patient, Mr Fred Jones, who attempted suicide after a poorly communicated diagnosis of terminal illness. Is Mr Jones also a part? Is he a 'member' of the ward? Does he too have to 'fit in'? What does he fit into? If the ward 'runs like clockwork', is he a 'component'? Does he have to 'work' at being a 'component-patient', and try to achieve 'good patient'-hood (i.e. nurse-preferred ward behaviour, cf. Johnson & Webb, 1994) in exchange for good nursing?

In the first place, then, we see that the ward is a system, an organised whole. In the second place, this system is functional; it does something special. The ward is the hospital's basic functional unit (Bopp *et al.*, 1996, p. 697). Functionally speaking, hospitals and wards exist because, like factories, they provide benefits of scale through the division of labour. Additionally, as with any organisation, joint actions coordinated are more productive than uncoordinated individual actions (Arrow, 1974, p. 53). The ward's job is to focus and coordinate the scientific, technological, economic, organisational and social authority resources of the health care system in its impact on hospital patients. So, as hospital employees assigned to wards, nurses are agents of a functional system, the last link in a chain of impersonal roles devised to control or defeat, with the greatest feasible efficiency, involuntary human malfunctioning. They may be jewels, but they must be jewels in a mechanism.[3]

If, as Adam Smith said, a system is an imaginary machine, the roles in an organisation can be played like the springs, cogs and levers that deliver the time-communicating service to the hands of a clock. Accurate and complete fulfilment of function as intended is all that is required. If one wanted to refer to an 'ideal type' mechanical caricature of a nurse, to a cog-like nurse whose sole intention was to carry out with the most complete distance and detachment his or her practical functions as organisationally prescribed,[4] one could coin the term 'warderly': the creature of the ward system as a technological device. Under the direction of his or her hierarchical superior,[5] the warderly carries out the part-activities (i.e. tasks) of the ward, leaving the superior to integrate the actions of each 'pair of hands' into the whole collection of tasks that make up the ward cycle (i.e. shifts). As the bottom link in the hierarchy of command the warderly looks up the chain of authority towards those who can hold him or her accountable for how well he or she has played a subordinate role as a ward operative.

This functional world is the one into which is brought the patient, the non-agent, the powerless one, the sufferer, Mr Jones. His deficient capacity for self-care means he needs the resources of the health service. Having lost his will to live also means that he is not best placed to negotiate his role in the hospital system; indeed, his illness may have made his identity so fragile that he cannot any longer play even his cardinal roles. But, although he is in hospital because he needs its functional resources, his functional deficits do not eliminate his human nature. Although impaired function-ally, he remains a person, an end in himself. It is because being ill or dis-turbed is not just having defective mechanical parts that a warderly is not enough. It is because being ill does not entail a loss of one's spiritual status as a human being that the patient needs nursing, with all the human attention that the word implies.

Fortunately, his nurse, Staff Nurse David Jones, understands his own ambiguity. He knows that, in order to meet the dual needs of Mr Fred Jones the patient, he has two sets of tasks – the organisational and the profes-sional. In his organisational role he has to find the politically acceptable point of equilibrium between the needs of the patient and the requirements of the ward authorities.[6] Politically Mr Jones by himself is in a vulnerable position – inpatients are 'out-powered'. His principal protection against being functionally objectified and processed like a baked bean (albeit with 'total quality') is his right (i.e. his acknowledged entitlement) to respect for his presumed personhood. This respect is still espoused as normative in our society, and still endorsed by the nursing profession. So Mr Jones needs not just the functional resources of the ward, but also the integrating (functional plus human) resources of his nurse. His entitlement to respect is valueless unless recognised by someone with the capacity to honour it. He needs a professional relationship.

As 'patient-nurse', therefore, one aspect of David Jones's professional task is to manage the ward environment on behalf of the patient. This is because there is more to caring for patients than looking after them as individuals: since Nightingale's *Notes on Nursing* the nurse has been enjoined to remember that the patient himself is not the whole of what must be managed if he is to be cared for. His nurse must also control the environment on his behalf, and this remains as true of the mental health nurse as of the general. To this end, Nurse Jones's professional right to command the functional resources of the ward is socially sanctioned, provided he be publicly recognised ('registered') as a fit and qualified person. But his mandate to manage the ward environment he acquires from Mr Jones.[7] Fred Jones is his client, to whom he feels himself professionally responsible. This means both that he is Mr Jones's agent in providing that care he would normally secure for himself, but also that Mr Jones remains the source of the authority which underpins that care.

Note that the patient does not confer his authority on the nurse; he or she is granted the exercise of it, to just that extent and for just that time which may be necessary. It is because Nurse Jones needs discretion to exercise his dual authority (with the patient, over the ward) that he is a professional, not because he has been delegated powers by his line manager. It's not my employer who makes me a professional, but my client. If I arrogate total authority to myself and reduce the client to dependence, I am acting as the apparatchik of the organisation as a processing plant, not as a professional.

The kind of care Mr Jones would secure for himself his nurse can only discover by relating to him person to person.[8] Especially in mental health nursing, the patient is often difficult to relate to as a person, so in this area nurses need a strong sense of personhood with which to call to the wounded or shocked personhood of their patients. Importantly, however, any nurse's capacity as a person is not merely an outcome of training. The spiritual, intellectual, moral and emotional resources necessary to relate to others as human beings grounded in our own personhood, we derive from our upbringing as one member of a society of persons. If we call such a client-relating agent a 'person artist',[2] we remind ourselves both that it is not something unique to nurses, and that this manner of being and relating, though manifested by individuals, is more than an individual skill; it is an achievement of the culture as a whole.[9] In the person of the nurse by the bedside stands an entire society which has, by producing and sustaining this human figure, decreed that none should suffer uncared for. Most frequently, the nearest hand in a chain of caring hands held out to over-come anguish belongs to a nurse. Even when we are not there, we are there, because nurses are us.

Ambiguity: personhood and the college classroom

The analysis thus far may be reinforced by extending it to another species of organisation. In broad terms the contradiction between a depersonalis-ing organisational environment and a professional ideology of personal relations within that environment was also characteristic of the classroom of the pre-Project 2000 (i.e. pre-1990) colleges of basic nurse training, at least in Scotland. The analytical ingredients differ: classroom instead of ward, learner instead of practitioner, teacher instead of charge nurse. Nevertheless, the constituents were similarly structured, with the same general kinds of relations prevailing, bringing with them too, unhappiness and wasted opportunities.[10]

Allow me once again to polarise into two ideal types: nurse tutor Anne Jones and student nurse Mary Jones. Nurse tutor Jones can be seen to be a hybrid; personally 'amphibious' between two worlds of meaning, although in practice restricted largely to one organisation, the school of nursing. Were she to become discouraged by her treadmill-like existence (from teaching the same material four times a year, for example), nurse tutor Jones might content herself with playing her organisational role mechanically in the prescribed way. The classroom teacher equivalent of the warderly is a matter-teacher. With very little time and a great deal of material to cover before the students went on the ward, the matter-teacher could be observed to aim for a point of equilibrium between the classroom needs of the students (such as their lack of familiarity with technical terms, forgetting of material covered in earlier modules, etc.) and the functional requirements of the imminent clinical area.

For teachers, trained to a largely uniform didactic approach by the college which then prepared most registered nurse teachers (RNTs), classes were marathons of informational down-loading, well-prepared acetates chasing each other across the OHP like swabs across the operating table. For students, classes were the equally gruelling construction of a file-library of notes and hand-outs, to be committed to memory at some future moment (ironically, often after five-sixths of the actual nursing experience to which the knowledge was relevant, i.e. just before the end of module exam).

Struggling to get out from behind this flood of information-giving it was often possible to discern the classroom counterpart of the patient-nurse. This was the nurse tutor Jones who wanted to be an educator rather than a kind of one-woman publisher; who had, from her own years of clinical experience, more important understandings with which to endow learners approaching their first day on a new ward than text-book information about psycho-medical conditions; who tried to prompt students into seeing (and valuing) their own individuality as reflected in the patients for whom they would soon be caring.

For Anne Jones as learner-tutor the classroom environment, (indeed, the college environment in general), appeared if anything less propitious for a meeting of persons than the average ward for her counterpart still in clinical practice. At least patients both knew that they needed personal care, and deeply appreciated what they actually got. Tied to the medical model for what they had to cover, RNTs were all but deprived of their most valuable teaching resource, their own experience of actual patients. Hence their learners, flash-matured from more recent clinical experience, silently but obviously relegated their would-be educators to a status inferior to their practice role-models on the wards. Barring personal problems or 'academic difficulties', few were available for 'extra-curricular' personal development. They hurried, 'open-eyedly anticipatorily self-socialised', towards a clearly-perceived future. As with all apprentices, the future was what they already knew, the reality of day-to-day work. As with apprenticeship in general, because they had worked hard to cover all possible eventualities, they did not expect to have to think[11] in the practice environment; hence all too often they could be seen sliding unawares from passive learner of files of matter to conforming instrument of the ward as a technological system, i.e. a warderly.[12]

So in fact, as the learner in the nursing college classroom, student nurse Mary Jones confronted a double ambiguity, one superimposed upon another, both damaging to her personhood. In the first place, though her educators may have wanted to be teachers of students, their organisational accountability was in effect for information successfully transmitted,[13] for exam passes; exams were failed because students were ignorant or forgetful, not because they remained personally immature. In the second place, Mary Jones's role-enactments in both the classroom and the ward were powerfully driven towards the functional by the way in which each setting was constructed and managed.[14] Both as an apprentice on the ward and as a student in college she was assessed on functional grounds. Encouragement of her personhood was left to the other (mostly very young) members of the (humanly highly solidaristic) cohort with whom she passed through the succession of functional hoops, with an occasional (but very significant) acknowledgement from a patient.

Ambiguity in perception, ambiguity in nursing practice

Nurses, then, operate in two distinguishable (but not separable) environments: the world of organisational roles, and the world of natural persons.[15] The nurse is a hybrid: an employee contracted to accept hierarchical authority, to act accountably in pursuit of the organisation's functional objectives; and also a professional committed subjectively to taking responsibility[16] for his or her exercise of the patient's delegated authority. Whereas to the organisation nurses are functional actors, patients look to them to be the mirror of their own personhood. In the ward situation, therefore, identities are uncertain: the patient, declared to be a whole, probably feels anything but a whole; the nurse, defined functionally as a part of the ward, is nevertheless supposed to function as a whole in relating to patients as individual persons.

I suggest that these identities are uncertain because here perceptions are not simple. The ward is not just a means for treatment, but also a means for meaning, a mechanism of perception; like a lens, it structures its objects and its actors (Rosenhan, 1973, p. 258). The nurse tends to be perceived differently (and therefore related to differently) by the different sets of actors with whom he or she works. As one is seen, so one sees oneself, so one defines oneself, so one becomes. Perceptions make self-conceptions. Because perceptions make self-conceptions, and therefore condition meaningful behaviour, perceptions are contested terrain. Of the competing perceptions in the ward, two predominate: that of the managers of the ward environment, and that of those who are managed by the ward environment. Hospital and patients struggle for primacy in the nurse's active self-constitution as a meaningful being.

Now here is the strange thing. As a fact about nursing this duality is inescapable – meaning that until I see it I am not seeing the ward (or the classroom) 'as they really are'. Yet in their practice good nurses do escape the duality; many patients do in fact get cared for as whole human beings in efficiently-run wards. Such nurses can overcome the contradictory either/or of organisational environments. How do they manage it? And what can we (including me) learn from them?

To explain their success it may help to speak in pictures. Fig. 8.1 shows the familiar picture of what can be interpreted either as a goblet or as two faces in profile. As the picture is drawn, to see a goblet you must see a white figure against a black ground; in order to see two faces in profile, you must see black figures against a white ground. Your choice of ground determines the figure you see, or vice-versa. The point of the exercise is to make clear that you can only see one or the other: seeing one as figure makes the other ground, and vice-versa. You can see either in quick succession to the other ('figure-ground reversal'); but you cannot see both simultaneously.[17]

With pictures of the figure-ground reversal type, while the two perceptions are reversible, each is coherent independently: you do see a cup, you do see two faces. To echo a phrase of a moment ago, they are not only distinguishable but separate. There is another class of pictures, however, where there are also two pictures; but instead of being reversible they are continuous. You cannot easily tell where one turns into the other. The drawings of M.C. Escher are perhaps the most famous examples; but the simple drawing reproduced as Fig. 8.2 makes my point more easily.

The ankle end of the jeans has three legs, but the thigh end has only two. The eye flicks back and forth trying to resolve the puzzle, but without success. Until, that is, we fix on the point of discontinuity, where we lose or gain a leg. Where is it? The artist has drawn a line (which I have marked A–B–C) which is common to both pictures, yet functions differently in each. At the ankle end (A and C) it creates a middle leg; while at the thigh end (B) it appears to be the inside edge of two legs, with no sign of any third leg. Indeed, if A and C had been joined to the bottom point of the top leg and to the top point of the bottom leg respectively, there would be no third leg.

How is this relevant to practising nurses? My suggestion is that the nurse who becomes a warderly views the organisational environment as we view the first picture: as two mutually exclusive separate cultures. Working with one entails a large neglect of the other. By contrast, nurses who escape the effects of the ward/person duality constitute the duality in a different way: not as either/or, not as figure or ground, but rather as a continuity, as a double world held together by an agent who can remain a person even when acting in role – a person artist.

Mature hospital nurses get the better of the structural-cultural contradiction in which they have to work through holding to a 'deep' approach[18] to nursing: acting out of their culturally-formed personal wholeness, through a ward role held in tension between organisational and professional requirements, towards sustaining the wholeness and self-care potential of the patient. The split, therefore, one can escape; but the tension inherent in the ward role – a role where one has to give personal care and to accept impersonal authority at the same time – it is the tension that one cannot escape. Not, that is, if one wishes to go on thinking of oneself as professional;[19] the warderly, in accepting the split as absolute, does escape the tension, and yields up the determination of his or her behaviour to the organisation and its demands.

Perhaps, therefore, rather than dualistically seeing (as the warderly does) the nurse as moving between two separable worlds, we should see nurse

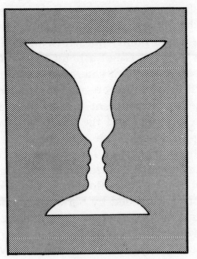

Figure 8.1

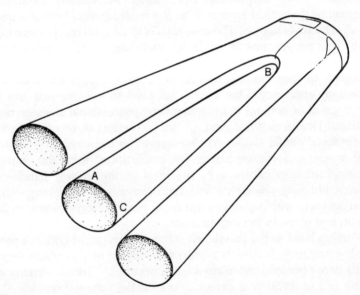

Figure 8.2

and ward as two opposing directions in one integral process: the nurse trying to project humane norms on to the ward, the ward 'trying' to map its efficiency norms on to the nurse. The relations of functional accountability and those of human responsibility run in opposing directions – the one away from the patient and towards organisational abstractions, the other from (yet still within) an organisation towards the patient as a human being. Seen like this, the relations are not mutually exclusive; they can be reconciled. From the struggle of functional and human can emerge a higher

good: a mature professional practitioner with power over the organisation's resources on the patient's behalf.

There is, therefore, a mid-point from which one can see both worlds. But
it is also an interior point. It is not a point you reach if you are merely
looking in order to see; it is a point where one sees differently because one
acts. It is called practice.[20] The person artist committed to a disciplined use
of themselves as a human 'instrument' in their professional work has to be
able to integrate the personal and the organisational in practice. Nurse
Jones has to manage himself as the interface of the inherent conflict of
interests between the managers of hospital resources and the patients.
Nurse tutor Jones has to manage herself in her role (Lawrence, 1979) in the
same way, because it is her organisational role which allows her to provide
the learning opportunities needed by her student clients. For both nurse
and tutor, success in the role is where the merely organisational role is
transcended[21] in favour of a professional role, even though this professional role is still actually played in the organisation. Managing oneself in a
role in these (and similar) settings means that one lives in tension. Though
challenging, it can be a satisfying way to live.[22]

If it is the case that mature practitioners are already the model for an
integrating dialectical approach to the contradiction between patient and
ward, why this chapter? The answer has to do with our present history. As
part of its programme to eradicate Victorian values, British government
policy has been subordinating the substantive objectives of public organisations to their procedural rules; their experienced quality to their
measured efficiency. One means adopted to achieve this has been the
substitution of general management for professional management in the
National Health Service. And, in turn, an effect of this has been that the
professional career ladder for the nurse has been reduced to two rungs:
staff nurse and charge nurse. By implication, therefore, nursing professionalism now contracts to the level of the trained hands-on practitioners. Nursing objectives and requirements above charge-nurse level
must compete with objectives and requirements from elsewhere, from both
within and outwith the organisation.

Nursing has lost the privileged status of a pyramid within a pyramid, of
a self-governing dominion within the empire of the health service, of a
multi-tiered profession within an organisation.[23] British nursing has come
to the end of its 50-year career as one of the national services,[24] and has
returned to its origins, as a single-layer expert profession. The ward is the
prime site for nursing's newly 'compacted' professionalism.[25] This means
the responsibility for securing professionalism in nursing now falls overwhelmingly on ward-level practitioners. No longer can hospital nurses go
along unquestioningly with decisions handed down from above, since
such decisions may have had no nursing criteria applied to them, even
though they may have been made by registered nurses. No longer can they
rely on their hierarchical superiors or professional leaders to protect their
professionalism from dilution or distortion, to help them even up the
imbalance of power between the organisation and the person. The ram-

parts and the baileys have fallen to the abstract forces of budgets and indicators; only the keep – the ward – remains.

This new situation demands from charge nurses and staff nurses a new vigilance on behalf of their patients; vigilance against a distorted version of themselves. Only practitioners sensitive to the patient and the ward as competing sources of meaning for their practice will maintain their professionalism into the new era. Secondly, only practitioners who know that their actions make social structures, who have recognised that in their practice they do overcome paradigms oriented to other goals, will be able to construct a philosophy-in-action which can withstand the ward as a machine. Organisations make the people who work in them, but the people who work in them have some power to make the organisation. To be professional is to own that power as a legitimate right, the authority to be exercised on behalf of the patients. So, while it is as detached lookers-on that we try to decide about the lines in the jeans drawing, it is as a committed agent with a power to make real that the nurse decides what kind of 'line' he or she is going to take on the ward. The artist in the drawing of the boundaries of inter-personal behaviour in the ward environment is the nurse. It is as practice-artists that nurses can transcend the apparent paradox of person and role by a principled professional self-management. And so can we.

Ambiguity in academic practice: where should we stand if we want to do more than look?

So can we? Who are 'we'? The answer to this question drives the argument a stage further than is customary in academic discourse, so it may help if I resume what I have been trying to say. I have argued: (a) that the contradictory quality of the nurse's experience is an outcome of the way the ward works as a dualistic system; and (b) that this dual nature of the ward as a nursing environment is inevitable, given its efficiency objectives as a technological form. The same is true of the classroom; its sheer economic efficiency dictates that, though other methods may supplement the classroom as a teaching technology, none can replace it. In each case, nurses' felt-ambiguity is a problem pre-set by the interaction of professional–personal ends with technological–organisational means (Scribner, 1986). Since nursing has only rarely been able to structure its work environments to achieve purely nursing objectives, such problematic work settings have long been a taken-for-granted fact of nursing life.

Such problematic work settings necessarily produce uncertain identities, both for workers and for clients, which largely derive from the capacity of the setting to structure perception. Observation shows, however, that many nurses have resolved the dualistic contradiction of the ward as an environment for nursing, and consistently meet the person-sustaining needs of their patients. They have the maturity to manage conflicting demands on them from clearly distinguishable life-worlds without being driven into behaviour appropriate to just one or the other.

Since this chapter has been a plea for awareness, it seems only fair to swivel the lens around and focus attention on us, the above-mentioned 'we', by which I mean academics. After all, if one argues for self-awareness, one ought to display it oneself. For it is not only nurses in clinical or nurse-teaching areas who have a crucial role in the formation of the profession of the future. Academic books and papers also structure perception. It is beyond question that nurses (and others like myself) working in academic institutions have acquired enormous power to guide the evolution of the profession, and to present it to public and politicians. This being the case, how much does the general thesis proposed for ward and classroom transfer to researchers? Is there a technological imperative distorting or squeezing out the personhood of researchers? Is the academic role free of structural contradiction? Are staff nurse Jones, nurse tutor Jones and student nurse Jones entitled to say: 'Are you sure, Dr Ryan, you are not living in a glass house?'

In other words, since I write in the style of an institutionalised academic, does my writing reconcile the system-needs of my organisation with the human needs of my presumed professional clients, my readers? How self-aware have I been in my relations with the academic writing life-world? Have I stood my ground in the interests of the personhood of my readers? Have I been as professional as those I have presumed to advise? Or have I been expecting my readers to pick up the cues from my passive moods, impersonal constructions, self-distancing general remarks, deferential references, to construct themselves as impersonal intelligences? To the last question I answer 'Yes'. To the previous four I answer 'Not much'. This suggests I need a new approach.

I would therefore now like to suggest that those who do research on nursing are just as likely to be amphibians as the nurses whose life-world they are trying to understand. For researchers, the technological structure which seeks to reduce them to cogs in the machine is also abstract, and therefore hard to see: it is the scientific project, a by-now-universal process of accumulating data in accordance with certain methodological proce-dures with the aim of overcoming, not just involuntary human mal-functioning, but every limitation to which Man feels subject. Its being an abstract rather than a concrete structure in no way lessens the imperious demandingness of the scientific project:

> 'The most redoubtable machines, perhaps, are not those that revolve or run... There are other kinds, not built of copper or steel, but of narrowly specialised individuals: I refer to organisations, those administrative machines constructed in imitation of the *impersonal aspects* of the mind.'
>
> (Valéry, 1963, p. 78, emphasis in original)

The real world institution which the scientific project has recently per-suaded to be its host is the university. Just as the hospital ward focuses upon persons deficient in their self-care capabilities all the resources of modern society, so the enquirer after knowledge will find the university a beautifully crafted machine for knowing. But insofar as knowing is equated with science, the university becomes limited: the limits, naturally, are those of the machine.

Fully paid-up subscribers to the scientific project have a difficulty with the notion of a person. The difficulty is that it is not divisible without remainder among the recognised academic disciplines. Contrast, for example, the tidily delimitable notion of 'role'. While role theory is a subtle and penetrating analytical tool, no personalist accepts that an individual is the sum of his or her role performances. There is an integrating core that persists between performances; persists, indeed, even without performances. As individual persons themselves, role theorists may admit this. But as academics they cannot escape from the fact that 'person' and 'role' construct different intellectual universes (Körner, 1971, p. 15), nor can they help us negotiate between the two without risking their standing in the academic community. The fundamental principle in the implicit contract subscribed to by all would-be scientists states that it is not scientific to be both in the landscape and viewing it at the same time: the only valid view is the spectator's (Holmes, 1990, p. 203). To say 'participant' is to say 'bias'.

Here our two pictures may again be worth many words. I would propose that Fig. 8.1 models the relationship of *difference*, as understood by devotees of the scientific project, between

(a) the universe of persons (including themselves, if and when they escape from thinking scientifically); and
(b) that theoretical universe within which is to be found the inner logic *both* of the scientific project *and* of formal-rational organisations (e.g. hospitals).

Perceptually, such a view puts us back in the perspective of figure/ ground reversibility. Identities are mutually exclusive. You see person *or* institutional role-player; person *or* scientist. When you focus on one, you lose the other. Approaches, too, are mutually exclusive. Adopt a 'properly scientific approach' and people (including the scientist implementing the approach) get reductively reconstituted as the objects and agents of the procedures of the disciplines. Scientific method is *proper* procedure, the procedures appropriate to objects as constituted by the scientific world-view, proper to agents as constituted by scientific language. Science speaks me, much as Apollo 'spoke' the Delphic oracle. Who I am matters not a jot, no more than did the individual priestesses who verbalised the utterings at Delphi. So: default on proper procedure, lose science-appropriate object – therefore no science. Mention yourself in the first person and 'object'-ivity vanishes.

Now I have already stated that I see the mature hospital nurse as potentially in the position of the double-duty line A–B–C in the jeans picture (Fig. 8.2), of being a signifier in two simultaneously existing signifieds, of having one meaning in one environment and a different meaning in the other environment – *but able to hold the two environments together, and therefore also the two meanings*. Fig. 8.2, therefore, presents us with a different way of looking. Certainly, one sees one or another version (two-legged or three-legged), but one also remains aware that there is a *whole* (trousers), that both options exist within the whole, and that there is continuity between the two versions. Figure 8.2, therefore, models a relationship of *tension*.

What then of ourselves? Which figure models the position of nursing academics, researchers, research funders, editorial committees? 'Ourselves' means that you must answer this question from your own experience. From my experience I judge that university nursing is closer to Fig. 8.1 than to Fig. 8.2, that we feel constrained to pursue 'objectivity' so as not to 'contaminate' our judgement with 'subjective' (therefore implicitly untrue) perceptions. But: do we assume that the nurse in his or her hospital organisation should be able to bridge those two realities – and as potential patients we do devoutly assume it[26] – while we in our organisations cannot, and should not? Are we therefore cogs and levers in thrall to the scientific project? Can we justly claim an emancipated autonomy equal to that of the patient–nurse? Or is the hospital nurse a privileged being, angelically at ease in both dispensations, able to shake off the trammels of depersonalisation that hold us fast?

I myself don't think we are as fast held by the trammels of depersonalisation as we pretend. Again, what is crucial is how we define the situation, which is something about which we do have a choice. If we construct a world from which we distance ourselves so as to put it to the question, then improper scientific behaviour does produce defective results, as discussed above. But what if we define it as a world to immerse ourselves in? Indeed, treat ourselves as worldlings who are essentially part of it, rather than alien Attenboroughs saucered in on scientific safari, soon to be saucered home again? The world is not just something we see, but is also somewhere we act. Anybody who has to act can escape a theory devised for looking. So, employing some such hermeneutic process as 'reflexive determination' (Maynard & Wilson, 1980, p. 293), we too may be able to find the equivalent of the common line in the jeans drawing: the point of transition from one universe to the other – which is also, therefore, where we create an integrated higher-order universe. This is the point where we must stand if we are not to feign impotence before the divine right of all-reducing mechanism; if we are to do justice to the world of our research subjects as a human world, one where the disciplined search for law-governed patterns of phenomena coexists with the acknowledgement that human 'phenomena' are uncompassable persons, ends in themselves.

And so I would suggest that, in university research as in hospital nursing, our practice is where we overcome dehumanising categories forged in science's long quest to objectify and subjugate nature. For academics, hands-on practice is writing: pursuing what may be true and sharing those fragments of truth we may believe we have found. Practice is process, not content. Writing is action, not theory: we are speaking through our hands, as it were therapeutically touching the eyes of readers rather than the skin of patients.

'The utterances of the self in practical activity are, for the most part, actions; [the self in practical activity] reveals itself in conduct.'

(Oakeshott, 1962, p. 211)

Speaking, and being spoken. As responsive academic practitioners, just as our fieldwork can turn up things which we were not looking for, so our writing can turn out things we didn't intend to say, which are nonetheless true and worth saying. However, if, out of fear that Big Academic will put me on a RAE-orientated drip of awareness-diminishing research, or transfer me to the locked ward of a teaching-only institution, I score out utterances which were soundly found and are ready to be said, then I am acting as an *acada-mechanic*, the academic fellow-creature of the hospital warderly, a task-oriented pair of hands at the word processor, a tractable intellectual operative cogging and levering in the system of the university as a technological form. Instead of actively pursuing truth, I have fallen passive victim to an organisation, a specialised machine. I fall victim because of the hold the theory of the machine already has over my consciousness. Indeed, in my practice, in my writing work (which includes reading the writing of others), I observe my academic superego policing the paragraphs, only too happy to don the role-robes of critical parent, thereby exerting the same *kind* of pressures towards mechanical practice as I have laboured to identify in nursing practice in ward and in classroom.

So, while this paper set out to advocate a leery watchfulness for would-be professional nurses in the handling of *their* depersonalising organisational environment, the-paper-as-practical-process has discovered that we researchers[27] are no less at risk of functioning as agents of a disempowering objectification of nursing practice. In both cases it is because the organisation can produce more tangible pleasure and pain to persuade us to accept its theory of itself and to 'en-role' in support of its procedures. Loyalty pays. But, if less tangible, there are fuller pleasures (and, indeed, sharper pains) than those which come to loyal role-players. Just as not every nurse is a warderly, so not every academic wishes merely to pile up methodologically pure data-bricks in the back-to-paradise tower of the grandiose scientific project. We can construct working in the university as a value commitment of a more-than-functional kind no less than does the person-artist in the hospital ward. Going beyond the functional means operating at a higher level of tension, of challenge, and, I hope, of satisfaction.

I conclude that we academics too must learn to stand at the inner point where we can serve both science[28] and human being. Just as nursing is a practice which cannot submit to the technological imperatives of the hospital, so nursing is also one of those university disciplines which cannot prostrate itself before scientific method. The university is not just a scientific institution; the hospital is not just a technological institution. Both are also humanistic institutions. They challenge us to humane thinking, humane acting. Ambiguity is of the essence.

Notes

1. For the purposes of the paper I have taken mental health nursing in hospital settings to be similar to general nursing with regard to the effect of the hospital as an organisation on the practice of the nurse.

2. As I have tried to raise similar issues before, a brief rehearsal in a note may protect the readability of this text. In earlier work (Ryan, 1985) I proposed a four-fold classification which recognised that not all 'professions' related to their clients as whole persons. Those which did (focusing their work on improving the overall spiritual, emotional, physical and social well-being of individuals) I thought could usefully be redefined as the *person arts*. These needed to be distinguished from:

   (a) those activities whose principal function was to make money for the organisation carrying them out;
   (b) those activities directed to benefitting society as a whole; and
   (c) those activities (sports, arts, learning) felt to have intrinsic value.

   That paper concerned itself with the particular needs of young entrants to the person arts for a professional education which was realistic about the human richness and organisational obstacles encountered when working with whole people. This paper is concerned with only one of the person arts, nursing; with nursing's most typical organisation rather than with the profession; and looks at practice rather than education. The question behind it remains the same as in 1984: how can professionals be enabled to respond better to problems which affect individuals as whole people?

3. In passing, it is good to recognise that the ward's modern *raison d'être* has more to do with efficiency than care.

4. The patient unable or unwilling to play the patient role may look to a nurse-person for support, only to find that the nurse has been taken over by the technical ward role. The nurse is object-ified by the *mere* role, just as the *too* clinical object-ifies the patient. Importantly, a patient's experience of being treated as a thing is often the corollary of his nurse's prior experience of being treated as an instrument. Instruments are non-reflexive means of action; they act but don't react; they effect change but remain unaltered themselves. Technologies instrumentalise. As Joseph Weizenbaum has said, 'when we grasp an artifact it grasps us'.

5. Much though we regret hierarchies, they are indispensable to the organisation of large systems. They provide control. But control can be of different kinds. It is legitimate to complain that many hospitals have persisted overlong with mechanistic models of control, although cybernetic models have been understood for many years. I have contrasted the command hierarchy, where the patient is at the bottom, with a 'support hierarchy', a cybernetic control hierarchy where the patient is at the top, in Ryan (1989b).

6. It seems to have long been the charge nurse's prerogative to decide where the point of equilibrium fell. Polarising for emphasis: for some charge nurses *patient needs* outweighed all but the most fundamental ward requirements (e.g. safety); for others, only when all the apparent *system needs* of the ward (down to e.g. tidyness) had been fully met could nurses address the non-functional needs of patients (e.g. conversation). Hospital nursing as bequeathed by Nightingale (reasonably enough, given the then ratio of trained to untrained staff) was a job and a half for Sister, half a job for everybody else. The

degradation of the staff nurse's work into tasks is perhaps the source of the extraordinary salience of the term 'work' (i.e. 'labour') in first-hand accounts of what they do by British nurses (compare the accounts in Melia (1987) with those in Olesen & Whittaker (1968)). It also, in my view, points up the urgency – if the possibility of *professional* practice for staff nurses is to survive – of the progression to primary nursing in British hospitals.

7.   If this is accepted, it entails that any development where unqualified staff do most of the hands-on nursing is regressive and anti-professional. The patient receiving direct care from someone without authority over the environment is not being nursed, in any post-Nightingale sense of the term.

8.   Donald Schön (1983, p. 41) has pointed out that standard techniques cannot be applied 'to a case that is not in the books'; for a unique case an understanding must be constructed, and, where the situation is problematic, that understanding must be reframed. In a specifically nursing perspective, Alfano (1985, p. 28) typifies the nurse's evaluation of the patient's needs as general and objective, as contrasted with the patient's own evaluation of his needs as specific and subjective.

9.   'Education, in its broad sense, is more comprehensive than schooling, since it encompasses all those processes through which a society's members are developed. Indeed, all institutions influence the development of persons working within, or affected by, them. Institutions are complex structures of actions and expectations, and to live within their scope is to order one's own actions and expectations in a manner that is modified, directly or subtly, by that fact... All institutions have an educational side, no matter what their primary functions may be.' (Scheffler, 1973, p. 139)

10. In Ryan (1988) I proposed that the real problem of the then pattern of nurse training was not the integration of theory and practice but accommodating the implications of wholeness in the first place. Because the powerful in our society now see these as impossible to accommodate, the less powerful are left to live out this failure as contradictions and stress in their lives, learning and practice.

11. 'Thinking is trying to make up for a gap in your education.' Gilbert Ryle (quoted in Schrag, 1987, p. 481).

12. 'Much of the problem in leading a child to effective cognitive activity is to free him from the immediate control of environmental rewards and punishments. Learning that starts in response to the rewards of parental or teacher approval or to the avoidance of failure can too readily develop a pattern in which the child is seeking cues as to how to conform to what is expected of him.' (Bruner, 1962, pp. 87–88)

13. Students are less dependent than patients, so psychologically suffer less from what they have not received. But I observed that many tutors suffered from what they had not given.

14. Paradoxically – and another reason why most students preferred the ward to college – they reportedly were able to achieve more individual discretion (and so could be more 'responsible'/professional) in the ward (especially when the ward was short of qualified staff, e.g. on night duty) than they could in college. I have attempted a systematic comparison of wards and classrooms as technological forms in *Professional organization as technology: the ward and the classroom compared*, a paper for the Department of Health and Nursing, Queen Margaret College, Edinburgh, October 1993.

15. I accept that personhood is not 'natural' but a product of culture. I also accept

that, as an understanding of the potential of human nature, it is historical, one not shared even by earlier ages of our own culture. Nevertheless it is something we now recognise to be (and therefore constitute as) an almost inevitable outcome of 'primary socialisation' (the experience of infancy and childhood). Hence 'natural'. By contrast, occupational role behaviours are the largely predetermined result of purposive learning programmes ('secondary socialisation') set up with specific aims and objectives by those who control the occupation.

16. That responsibility for others may be largely a subjective commitment on the part of workers as persons does not mean that efficiency-maximising organisations do not benefit from its presence in the organisation. Kenneth Arrow sees the exercise by professionals of responsibility as a means whereby organisational authority can be protected from unnecessary error. 'Responsibility is a system where authority performs its functional role but is subject to corrective action by its subjects,' (Arrow, 1974, p. 65). 'The basic deficiency of irresponsible authority from the functional viewpoint is the likelihood of unnecessary error ... where information is available somewhere in the organisation but not available to or not used by the authority' (1974, pp. 73–74). 'Authority may be wrong in contexts where a corrective mechanism [i.e. professional expertise] is potentially available' (1974, p. 75). It is good to have the suggestion that the the cheapest staffing mix may not be the most efficient coming from a Nobel prize-winner in economics.

17. A similar and most helpful distinction, between 'focal' and 'subsidiary' awareness, is made by Michael Polanyi (1958, pp. 55–57).

18. The distinction between a 'deep' and a 'surface' approach to work I take from the studies of Marton *et al.*, summarised in Entwistle (1987).

19. On this definition, some charge nurses may well be incapable of ever being truly professional, while some unqualified nursing aides may be professional from day one. Almost any patient could confirm this. But remember that another definition of professional requires that they can control the environment in the patient's interests. Aides (usually) cannot do this. To save misunderstanding, note well that 'warderly' is not a synonym for auxiliary/aide; it is not a property of junior rank, but defines an approach.

20. I present the idea of nursing as a practice-led profession in Ryan (1989b).

21. Going beyond the role can lead the reflective carer to see better how her work and the institution inter-relate, and even to the foundation of new kinds of institution. Cicely Saunders built the hospice because hospital wards denied her the relationships with the dying she believed to be appropriate to their needs (du Boulay, 1984, pp. 54–59, 78–87).

22. It is because life on this frontier is one of constant responsible decision-making that nurses are professionals, though their professionalism may be hindered by a manager who cannot or will not build a person-sustaining practice. Ward leadership is crucial for the human quality of a ward. The failure of Project 2000 to integrate the new learner preparation programmes with staff and organisational development programmes in the practice areas may result in the continuation of much sub-professional nursing – if by super-prepared practitioners. But such failures are just further symptoms of the declining capacity of our polity to integrate anything at all and need separate, lengthy, treatment (i.e. beyond that in Ryan, 1989b).

23. The Salmon Report (1969) led to the most extended structures for nursing self-management.

24. The service/profession distinction is introduced in Ryan (1989a).
25. Introduced in my 'Hierarchy in the health service and compacted professionalism in nursing: a historical view', paper to a joint meeting of the Departments of Nursing Studies and of Social Policy, University of Edinburgh, Edinburgh, November 1993.
26. The possibility that each of us may come to be a patient of a nurse we have helped to form takes the discussion beyond reflexivity, to justice. What right have I to hope for a mature, person-regarding nurse when I am reduced by illness if, while I am well, I have not fought for person-respecting attitudes and policies in that part of the culture in which I work?
27. For an emblematic experience of an academic researcher in the mental health context being led by a patient to desist from her depersonalising role-robotics, see Bellaby (1972).
28. I have not been arguing that the scientific project should be evicted from universities, though it is an argument that can be made, as for instance by Nicholas Maxwell (1984, p. 153: 'For I am advocating nothing less than that the basic aims and methods, the whole character, of the academic enterprise be changed'). I am saying that we may have presumed its principles to be normative for university disciplines in general, which for nursing would, in my understanding of what nursing aspires to be, entail a derogation of its character as a humane inter-personal practice, as a person art.

Acknowledgements

The research from which this paper derives was carried out while I was Research Fellow, Evaluation of the (Scottish) 1982 Scheme of Basic Nurse Education and Training Project (Project Director: Professor P. Prophit), University of Edinburgh Department of Nursing Studies, 1986–1989. The paper does not claim to represent the views of the funder, the director, or the host department.

References

Alfano, G. (1985) Whom do you care for? *Nursing Practice* **1**, 1.
Arrow, K.J. (1974) *The Limits of Organization*. Norton, New York.
Bellaby, B. (1972) A sociologist joins in. In *A Hospital Looks at Itself: Essays from Claybury* (E. Shoenberg ed.). Cassirer, Oxford, pp. 264–270.
Bopp, J.H., Ribble, D.J., Cassidy, J.J. & Markoff, R.A. (1996) Re-engineering the State Hospital to promote rehabilitation and recovery. *Psychiatric Services* **47** (7), 697–701.
Bruner, J.S. (1962) The act of discovery. In *Knowing: Essays for the Left Hand*. Belknap Press, Cambridge, Massachusetts, pp. 81–96.
du Boulay, S. (1984) *Cicely Saunders: Founder of the Modern Hospice Movement*. Hodder and Stoughton, London.
Entwistle, N. (1987) A model of the teaching-learning process. In *Student Learning: Research in Education and Cognitive Psychology* (J.T.E. Richardson, M.W. Eysenck & D. Warren Piper eds). Society for Research into Higher Education and Open University Press, Milton Keynes, pp. 13–28.
Holmes, R. (1990) Person, role and organization: some constructivist notes. In *The Theory and Philosophy of Organizations: Critical Issues and New Perspectives* (J. Hassard & D. Pym eds). Routledge, London, pp. 198–218.

Johnson, M. & Webb, C. (1994) The power of social judgement: struggle and negotiation in the nursing process. Unpublished manuscript, University of Huddersfield, Huddersfield.

Körner, S. (1971) *Abstraction in Science and Morals*. Cambridge University Press, Cambridge.

Lawrence, W.G. (1979) A concept for today: the management of oneself in role. In *Exploring Individual and Organizational Boundaries: A Tavistock Open Systems Approach* (W.G. Lawrence ed.). Wiley, Chichester, pp. 235–249.

Maxwell, N. (1984) *From Knowledge to Wisdom: A Revolution in the Aims and Methods of Science*. Blackwell Science, Oxford.

Maynard, D.P. & Wilson, T.P. (1980) On the reification of social structure. In *Current perspectives in social theory. Volume 1* (S.G. McNall & G.N. Howe eds). JAI Press, Greenwich, CN, pp. 287–322.

Melia, K. (1987) *Learning and Working: The Occupational Socialization of Nurses*. Tavistock, London.

Oakeshott, M. (1962) *Rationalism in Politics*. Methuen, London.

Olesen, V. & Whittaker, E. (1968) *The Silent Dialogue: A Study of the Social Psychology of Professional Socialization*. Jossey Bass, San Francisco.

Polanyi, M. (1958) *Personal Knowledge: Towards a Post-Critical Philosophy*. Routledge and Kegan Paul, London.

Rosenhan, D.L. (1973) On being sane in insane places. *Science* **179**, pp. 250–258.

Ryan, D.P. (1985) The professional and the personal: are they incompatible? In *Accountable Autonomy: Perspectives in Professional Education* (S. Goodlad ed.). SRHE Annual Conference 1984. Society for Research into Higher Education, Guildford, pp. 56–75.

Ryan, D.P. (1988) *Theory and Practice in the Modular Scheme*. Evaluation Project Discussion Paper No. 2. University of Edinburgh, Department of Nursing Studies, Edinburgh.

Ryan, D.P. (1989a) *The Student and the Cadet: Models of the Learner in the British Professions*. Evaluation Project Discussion Paper No. 3. University of Edinburgh, Department of Nursing Studies, Edinburgh.

Ryan, D.P. (1989b) *Project 1999: The Support Hierarchy as the Management Contribution to Project 2000*. Evaluation Project Discussion Paper No. 4. University of Edinburgh, Department of Nursing Studies, Edinburgh.

Scheffler, I. (1973) Moral education and the democratic ideal. *Reason and Teaching*. Routledge and Kegan Paul, London.

Schön, D.A. (1983) *The Reflective Practitioner: How Professionals Think in Action*. Temple Smith, London.

Schrag, F. (1987) The classroom as a place for thinking. In *Thinking: The Second International Conference* (D.D. Perkins, J. Lochhead & J. Bishop eds). Erlbaum, Hillsdale, New Jersey, pp. 475–486.

Schumacher, E.F. (1979) *Good Work*. Jonathan Cape, London.

Scribner, S. (1986) Thinking in action: some characteristics of practical thought. In *Practical Intelligence: Nature and Origins of Competence in the Everyday World* (R.J. Sternberg & R.K. Wagner eds). Cambridge University Press, Cambridge, pp. 13–30.

Valéry, P. (1963, original French edition 1925) Remarks on intelligence. In *History and Politics*. Translated by D. Folliot and J. Mathews. Collected Works of Paul Valéry, Vol. 10. Routledge and Kegan Paul, London: pp. 72–88.

Wittgenstein, L. (1952) *Philosophical Investigations*. Translated by G.E.M. Anscombe. Basil Blackwell, Oxford.

9 Therapeutic Mental Health Nursing in the Acute In-Patient Setting: Mission Impossible?

Duncan Tennant

Introduction

This chapter is an account of the work of a group of mental health nurses in an acute in-patient department of a Scottish psychiatric hospital from the mid 1980s to the present day. It is written from the perspective of a mental health clinical nurse specialist with responsibility for the development of interpersonally-focused approaches to mental health nursing during this period.

My focus will be on the development of the group therapy programme in the wards in question. This is only one apect of what these nurses do (and it is only one part of my own role) but it is probably the one in which the tensions and contradictions of our work surface with the greatest frequency and intensity.

Readers requiring definitive answers about what mental health nursing is all about are advised to read no further. The chapter is 'more of a journey than a destination'. This does not mean that I have no firm beliefs about what is helpful to patients, or what mental health nurses should be doing. It is more that these beliefs change all the time and that there are dangers associated with 'firmness of belief' in a field which is relatively incomprehensible.

Not the least of these dangers is that 'the simplistic adoption of one discourse as the only "true" one will render impossible the task of unravelling the complexities of people's experiences of themselves and others.' (Banton *et al.*, 1985, p. 27)

The group room: 1995

Surveying the group therapy room. A carelessly discarded empty box of Kleenex and an uneven circle of empty chairs. The dead campfire of the last meeting of the group. It is difficult to believe that the best part of a decade separates it from the first one, though the battle-hardened reflection in the one-way mirror suggests twice as long as this. The result of high mileage as opposed to age. How much of my difficulties have been self-inflicted I am not sure. In retrospect, I probably arrived here with a level of 'street-wisdom' on a par with that of Bambi.

Prior to coming here I had been in the fortunate position of working in a department of adolescent psychiatry where interpersonal approaches were valued, as was the concept of the nurse as therapist. I considered myself equally fortunate to be given the responsibility of developing these approaches in adult psychiatry in the capacity of clinical nurse specialist. It was shortly before taking up this new position that I first realised that my luck was about to change, and it is at this point that my account begins.

Conference room: mid 1980s.

I was in the hospital conference room presenting four case studies involving the successful outcome of a family therapy approach to the treatment of anorexia nervosa. The audience consisted mainly of psychiatrists and I was somewhat taken aback by their reaction to what I was saying.

The content of my presentation was littered with disease-oriented terminology such as 'interpersonal psychopathology' and 'dysfunctional parental subsystem' – not exactly mainstream psychiatry, but I thought I was talking their language.

The approach I was describing was based on the premise that certain types of communication patterns in families led to psychosomatic symptoms in one individual family member. The model had been tested in the tradition of 'hard science'. Men in white coats had taken blood samples to measure changes in the free-fatty-acid levels of patients during therapy, in order to prove the link between these physiological changes and the dysfunctional communication which was taking place. A fine example of pioneering work in the medicalisation of human conflict and distress. It should not have been offensive to a medical audience, yet the climate in the room was one of unrest.

Question time. A psychiatrist asked whether I had considered that the successful outcome in these cases was due to the fact that the patients were not 'truly anorexic'. Her conviction was not swayed by my reminder that each case had previously been deemed to fulfil the DSM III diagnostic criteria by the psychiatrist who made the initial assessment. My patience wore thin. I wondered aloud what the overall rate of mis-diagnosis might be if her contention was correct (realising the recklessness of these words too late to stop myself from uttering them).

The discussion proceeded in a downhill trajectory from this point onward. Voices were raised and in the debate which followed there was little exploration of the issues at stake. I skilfully defended my point of view (as did my opposition) but the emphasis of both parties was on just that – defence.

I felt like an intruder who had moved into a restricted area – that my attempt to widen the frontier of understanding had instead degenerated into an acrimonious skirmish with the border guards.

In the struggle to make sense of this encounter, I had great difficulty in seeing things from the medical perspective. My thoughts were of Andrew Scull's chilling account of doctors locating mental illness in the brain in order to claim jurisdiction over it, and of doing so on a far from scientific basis. They had argued that physical treatments 'worked'. The uncritical faith in this contention was exemplified by Murray Cox, who achieved 'improvement' in patients by suspending them in mid-air and rotating them at 100 times per minute. The idea of the conscious choice of sane behaviour on the part of the patient (to avoid further rotation) was missing from the analysis of what 'worked'.

The limitations of their paradigm had survived the onslaught of Laing (1961, 1967), Szasz (1963, 1972) and Cooper (1978) who pointed out the role of psychiatry in the removal of mental health from social context and *vice versa*. Their authoritative position remained undented despite the charges filed by later commentators (Busfield, 1986, Miller & Rose, 1986) that psychiatry had as much to do with social control as it did with cure.

An often-cited example was the removal, in 1973, of homosexuality as a category of mental illness, an event described by Johnstone (1989, p. 245) as '... perhaps the most spectacular instant cure achieved by modern psychiatry, when homosexuality was dropped as a mental illness category and millions of people "recovered" overnight'.

A common thread of these critiques was the ambiguous nature of psychiatry, in that it played a central role in providing a cure for mental health problems, while at the same time shaping the way in which these problems are defined. Critical awareness of this ambiguity is conspicuously absent from psychiatrists' accounts of their work.

The family intervention I had described to my medical colleagues 'worked' but the complex interpersonal focus of the model (and the fact that is was being delivered by a nurse) resulted in a relocation of the goal posts of a definition of what works. My conclusion was that I had asked much of them. I was suggesting a paradigm shift which they could not permit themselves to make, regardless of whether or not it was framed in medical terminology. The words of David Cooper (1978, p. 157) rang in my ears:

> 'As the medical attitude always seeks the concrete, the substantial, the locatable, the idea of finding supposedly pathological processes, going on as it were, in the empty spaces between entities, is disturbing to the medical consciousness: everything in the field of investigation becomes flux, contradiction, the negation of negation and the vertiginous spiralling of endless meta-levels of discourse.'

My own profession had, in contrast, been 'vertiginously spiralling' for decades in terms of its own conceptual activity. Nurse theorists had espoused an interpersonal focus, beginning with the work of Render (1947) and Peplau (1952), and this was reflected in the 1950s nursing research activity, two-thirds of which constituted studies of interpersonal aspects of mental health nursing (Sills, 1977).

This research emphasis continued throughout the 1960s and the interpersonal relationship research interest was extended to encompass environmental and systems issues. The result of this widening of the scope was that the psychiatric nursing theory and research agenda became increasingly complex. This complexity is conveyed by Sills (1977):

'It is as if a person needs three sets of lenses to view the phenomena. One set of lenses sharply defines the individual; one set sees the relationship; the third set scopes the larger system. However, if all that the wearer of these tri-focal lenses sees is consequently blurred, then where is he? Perhaps it takes practice to use the trifocals and the headaches are only temporary.'

By the 1980s, the enormity of the task of developing a conceptual base for mental health nursing was summed up by Collister's (1988) suggestion: 'It could be that a meta-paradigm of nursing would include all models of nursing currently in existence, all those yet to be developed and published, and all other theory which provides knowledge for nurses in practice'. Reed (1987) was proposing a plan for the development of a theory for psychiatric nursing which embedded no less than seven nursing models in the four domains of nursing's meta-paradigm.

The task of developing nursing practice driven by such a wide theoretical agenda seemed to me quite impossible given the restrictive nature of the prevailing medical paradigm. In view of the clash which had just occurred, I decided that my goals required a little downward adjustment in terms of ambition.

One of my earliest observations was that the acute inpatient wards did not have a group therapy programme. In view of Yalom's (1983) recently published blueprint for such a programme, and his research review suggesting it was difficult to justify the effectiveness of wards which operated without such a programme, this seemed a good place to start.

I discussed this with various members of staff and it was agreed that I would attend ward rounds with a view to offering assistance with this and other deficits in the treatment programme. My first visit to a ward round did little to re-ignite my already dampened enthusiasm. The meeting was directed by a psychiatrist and most of the discussion was about biophysical causality and pharmacological intervention. I was surprised to see that a pharmacist was present to offer any required advice on the various potions which were the mainstay of treatment.

I had come from the inpatient adolescent unit where it was highly unusual for patients to be on drugs at all. (I was mercifully spared the knowledge that 10 years later the reverse would be the the case and that by 1995 the pharmacist would be attending the adolescent ward round like clockwork.) I was also used to more friction than I was witnessing here. The adolescent team meeting often crackled with affect as staff members fought to have their conflicting theoretical views heard by their equally vociferous colleagues. There was no evidence of a struggle here. No one seemed to take offence at anything.

The agenda of the meeting did include issues other than medication but the handling of these issues was on a common-sense basis rather than theoretically informed. Psychological interventions seemed to be carried out with staff needs in mind rather than those of the patients. Staff from various disciplines were allocated appropriate tasks and every one seemed to compete for medical endorsement of their work rather than working collaboratively to provide alternatives to the predominately biophysical conceptualisation of problems.

The nurses were fluent in the language of biophysical psychiatry and they spoke it with no trace in their accent of the afore-mentioned nursing theory. After the first 10 minutes, I heard little of the discussion as my thoughts drifted to Towell's (1975, p. 86) description of instructions given by a doctor at the top of the nursing notes with regard to 'General attitude to be adopted toward patient ... '. The back page of the record was headed 'Nursing notes: to be read and initialled at least once a week by doctor', ensuring that the nurses' records were regularly audited by the doctor. Other unwelcome memories of nurses doing little other than executing medically prescribed treatment followed thick and fast (see, for example, Cormack, 1983).

My impression, from discussion with various members of staff was that the medical staff viewed anything resembling a psychodynamic approach as dangerous, particularly if it took place in a group. Since these views were not expressed openly at the ward meetings, I decided, in collaboration with the ward nursing staff, to commence the group and inform the medical staff of the starting date.

The first meeting came and went with the patients in universal agreement that it had a been a useful experience for them. The second meeting shed more light on the impact that the venture had had on the wider system of the ward. It began with a review of the previous day's meeting and this was followed by comments about the unusual number of medical staff who had been on the ward the previous evening after the group had finished at 5 pm.

It eventually transpired that most of the patients in the group had been seen by a psychiatrist in the 24 hours between the first and second meeting. It also transpired that the group had been on the agenda at each of these interviews. Their feedback to the medical staff was overwhelmingly positive. The idea of this sudden intensive medical input as anything other than coincidence did not linger long in my thoughts. What difference did it make? If there were concerns for the safety of the patients then it was correct that this scrutiny took place. Besides, I had cause for satisfaction with the oucome of this scrutiny. The undeniable demonstration of consumer confidence was a major step towards obtaining security clearance for the group.

The ward round that week proceeded in the usual way. The first patient's medication was reviewed. The psychiatrist in charge prescribed the regime for the next 7 days and then added 'I understand that she has been attending the group. This of course is the treatment of choice in her case. It is important that she continues to attend.'

I could not help but admire the deftness with which he had relocated the goal posts. In the space of 48 hours the group had been turned from a highly dubious nursing venture into a medically-prescribed intervention. I was shocked at my own reaction to this. It was not with anger but relief that I had made it past the border crossing and had come through customs with a controlled substance.

During the initial period of quarantine, I awaited further medical scrutiny and a campaign to undermine the credibility of the group. The strategies used by biophysically-oriented medical directors to quell psychotherapeutic invasion of inpatient turf were well documented (Yalom, 1983). I knew what to expect.

As time passed it became clear that no such campaign was going to materialise and in retrospect I realise that there was no requirement for it. The war was already won. The ward remained diagnostically-driven and the introduction of an alternative approach did not constitute a change in driver. There were a few minor skirmishes but these usually involved very junior medical staff. The more experienced psychiatrists actively endorsed the venture and encouraged the patients to make use of it.

Shortly afterwards I was asked by a consultant psychiatrist to set up similar groups in another acute ward. (He withdrew the request several weeks later due to his discovery that the ward nursing staff were totally against the idea.) More recently the response of one psychiatrist to the introduction of ward groups led by nurses was that they could have the patients abseiling down the side of the building if they wished, as long as it did not require input from the medical staff.

In retrospect, I view the psychiatrists' earlier apprehension as more about the safety of patients and the nurses' role in ensuring it, than about a threat to their power base. The decision on the level of observation of patients has major implications for the deployment of nursing staff. This decision is often one which is made by medical staff and one around which conflict over what nurses should be doing crystallises.

On occasion, several patients are deemed to require the constant accompaniment of a nurse. The result of this is that nursing resources are taken up with this task, to the detriment of therapeutic activity such as group meetings. A colleague in one of the wards has referred to this as 'man-to-man marking'. (For those unfamiliar with the game of soccer, this is a tactic whereby the more creative players of the opposing team are closely policed, thus negating the threat that they pose. Their policing responsibilities also keep more creative players in the nursing team out of mischief.)

This is one of a number of tensions which render the attainment of therapeutic nursing practice impossible in acute inpatient units. Fuller explication of these tensions will require a return to the group room.

The group room: 1995

The chairs now form a neat circle and the box of Kleenex Professional Tissues is in a more accessible location. We are about 5 minutes behind schedule. The ward is very busy and it is, of course, unreasonable to expect two nurses to be available for the duration of the group. Three patients are on 'close observation' and most of the others are either very unwell or meet the criteria for allocation to the 'demanding' category.

I should be surprised when the two nurses arrive with nine patients, including those on close observation, but I am not. The charge nurse has the tactical awareness which comes only with the experience of many previous campaigns in which her team has fought back from the brink of relegation. She is using a variation of 'zonal defence'. Instead of abandoning the group, she gets the close observation patients to take part. Since they are in the same room, it actually saves nursing resourses for the duration of the session. More importantly, it allows the patients to address the difficulty imposed by being on close observation, and it allows both nurses and patients to address directly other impediments to establishing a productive relationship. The image of their predecessors portrayed over the last half century is one of unmitigated failure to do so.

An early example is John's (1961) picture of the 1950s mental health nurse 'bumper-swinging' in the ward sitting room (to keep the floor immaculate, the nurse sedated and the patients lined around the walls). 'When you're polishing you're not thinking, and that's the idea,' explained one of the subjects in John's study, adding the final brushstroke to a grotesque caricature of the nurse keeping busy to keep his distance. ('Bumper swinging' refers to the characteristic floor polishing style adopted by attendants or nurses, as seen, for example, in the film of Kesey's *One Flew Over the Cuckoo's Nest*.)

In the three decades to follow, there was little evidence to suggest any change in this image. Wing and Brown (1970) found social interaction between nurses and patients to be rare, and that patients followed a routine which met staff needs rather than *vice versa*. Towell (1975) reported patient 'disturbance' being viewed as an interruption of the nurses' routine rather than a focus for intervention. Cormack's (1976) study suggested that the principal activity of nurses was the observation and monitoring of patients' progress rather than therapeutic interaction. The 1980s research offered little to suggest that a more pleasing portrait was evolving (Powell, 1982; Cormack, 1983; Clinton, 1985).

The nurses and patients present in the group this morning inhabit an environment similar to that occupied by their ancestors. The impediments to therapeutic nurse–patient interaction are as formidable now as they were at any time over the last half century. A strong argument can be made that the tension which exists between the nurses' custodial responsibilities, and their role as therapists, is of such magnitude that the two roles cannot co-exist.

Porter (1992) suggested of nurses: 'As long as they are given the responsibility for institutional order, their therapeutic relationship with patients will be compromised. Therapy depends upon social proximity while order depends upon social distance'. The same author pointed out that nurses are more likely to face retribution for failures in their custodial responsibities than for failures in their therapeutic ones, particularly when the safety of patients is at stake, and this is certainly true in the case of the nurses present in the group this morning. This tension between custody and therapy is an ever-present agenda item in the group sessions. I no longer view it as something which gets in the way of the 'work' of the group. I believe that for much of the time it *is* the work of the group.

For example, today's meeting begins with a barrage of complaints from the patients about the treatment they have been receiving on the ward. They complain that they are not understood by the staff, that staff do not spend enough time talking to them, that it is an ordeal to approach the nurses' station for assistance, and that they do not receive enough information or consultation about their treatment.

A participant observer, witnessing the same conversation taking place in the ward sitting room, would probably be building a picture of the worst aspects of psychiatric institutions. He could fill his notebook more quickly than the nurses could reach the floor polisher. My own 'notebook' is recording a different picture. One major difference about the conversation I am witnessing here is that the ward staff are hearing the complaints directly from the patients. They do not require the services of a researcher to unearth the information for them. Secondly, the nurses are viewing such 'disorderly conduct' not only as an indication of a healthy ward environment, but also as an indication that the group is properly focused on one of the most relevant tasks faced by both themselves and the patients.

Some of this morning's complaints are news to them – these can be investigated further and solutions can be sought. Some are unresolvable, and in such cases an explanation for this state of affairs can be forwarded. Some of the complaints are distorted or inaccurate and the meaning of these distortions or inaccuracies can be explored.

In this regard, the group can be an important window for the understanding of the wider system of the ward. This is not a new idea and group therapists in inpatient units have long been aware of its potential. For example, Kibel (1987) capitalised on Levine's (1980) conceptualisation of the group as a *'milieu* biopsy' and provided evidence that data generated in the group can be utilised by the wider system (the ward) to great benefit, provided the therapist can cultivate a relationship with administrative staff which is conducive to exchange of this information. Since the therapists in this morning's group *are* key participants in the administration of the ward they are in a much more suitable position to make use of these data.

In dealing with these difficulties in their relationships with nurses and the nature of the ward environment, patients face directly some of the interpersonal concerns which may have precipitated their hospitalisation. Peplau (1994) suggested that: 'The major work of professionals, especially psychiatric nurses, is defined by the nature of the struggle that patients must make to know and to overcome their difficulties in living with people outside the hospital'.

Much of the work of the group is concerned with knowing and overcoming the same difficulties in living with people *inside* the hospital. If they can complete this task, then they will be better prepared to deal with similar interpersonal difficulties outside the hospital. Patients are viewed as having to cope with a series of 'adaptive tasks' (Rutan *et al.*, 1988) related to their stay on the ward (such as coping with hospitalisation, staff, other patients; separation from family) and with a number of 'in group' tasks (such as trusting others, bearing discomfort, monitoring personal boundaries, and saying good-bye as they reach the end of their stay). In dealing with these tasks, patients use their habitual defences and these are observable in the 'here and now'. Although the understanding of these defences is viewed as important, the work which takes place in the group has as much to do with emphasising strengths as with detecting psychopathology.

The work of the nurses is to provide the conditions necessary for patients to achieve these 'in group' tasks. The interpersonal difficulties which manifest themselves on the ward are turned into opportunities to make sense of and master relationship difficulties outside the ward.

The same approach is applied to all of the other contradictions and tensions faced by both nurses and patients attempting to work together constructively. One such tension surfaces this morning as a patient gives glowing testimony to the drug which has transformed her life. She seems not to consider relevant the fact that she has made significant adjustments in her relationships with others, and that she has regularly participated in individual and group sessions with nursing staff.

On hearing her speak, my initial thought is of Lego's (1992) story about a patient who embarked on various drug trials and reported to a nurse: 'It was as though I was at the bottom of the ocean, cut off from air, light and life itself. The medication acted as a giant crane that came down and slowly lifted me up to the surface and I was alive again'. The nurse replied, 'That's wonderful, you were taking the placebo'.

In previous years, this thought would have lingered a while longer, or been replaced by thought of another anomaly, for example, of the widespread use of an antidepressant, after clinical trials showed it to be marginally less effective than the placebo (Mintz, 1964). I would not have been happy about talk of medication in this room. It interfered with 'proper work' in the group. The group was supposed to focus on enabling patients to take control of their lives. Medication was external to their control. I would not have given it houseroom.

These days I see the tension inherent in the simultaneous use of medication and talking therapies as 'grist for the mill'. Currently, group therapy as the sole treatment is unusual in any setting. In a survey of 143 group therapists in the USA, Stone *et al.* (1991) found that two-thirds of therapists included medicated patients in their ordinary outpatient groups and that 37% of the patients treated by these therapists were taking medication. In inpatient units, 'talking therapy' uncontaminated by drug treatment is even less common.

Not only is this a tension we must live with: it is one which can be turned to therapeutic advantage if we allow it to darken the door of the therapy room. My energies are now consumed with the search for integrative links between drug treatments and talking therapy, such as those provided by Zaslav and Kalb (1989):

'For patients with very disabling interpersonal pathology, medicines often represent hope for a recovery somehow accomplished without messy human entanglement. The group therapist inhabits a setting which places a premium on precisely this experiential and interpersonal data. Far from being an unprofitable area of attention and inquiry, we believe that in clinical practice this material may represent one of the most important windows available for a successful understanding of our group members.'

By adopting this approach we are attempting to facilitate the fruitful co-existence of two diametrically opposed vehicles of change (biophysical and psychotherapeutic), and this is not easy to achieve. These vehicles frequently collide in the group and such occasions require swift, thoughtful intervention at the moment of impact to ensure that the bodywork of neither is dented.

This morning's collision is handled well. The charge nurse redirects the traffic appropriately and the discussion moves on to exploration of the meaning that medication has for each member of the group. Unfortunately, the flow is interrupted by a patient requesting permission to leave the group. It is his first meeting and he has heard enough to convince him that it is a waste of time. He is anxious and wants to go back to the ward for a cigarette.

The charge nurse looks as if she would like to join him and I can hardly blame her. It is not yet lunch time and she is facing her third quintessential mental health nursing paradox. She has heard many patients say the same thing in their first meeting. Those who can be persuaded to persevere usually go on to benefit greatly after negotiating this initial hurdle. Her response could begin with: 'In my experience ... ', but these words do not fit well with the collaborative relationship she would prefer.

Her problem is one which has been well documented by nurse theorists over the past four decades, beginning with Render's (1947) view that the patient's refusal to accept treatment was the point at which psychiatric nursing intervention really began.

Travelbee's (1969, p. 149) advice on the matter was: 'The ill person, in effect, is *told that he is to participate*. As stated, a patient may become frightened or overwhelmed by this approach but the structure of the approach and *the fact that he has no choice can be helpful and comforting*' (emphasis added).

The words hardly sit comfortably with the 1990s language of collaboration and empowerment but Travelbee also had a point. If the patient leaves the room at this stage he may close the door on a valuable opportunity. The current thinking in the group therapy literature is that gentle pressure to participate is necessary as a demonstration of caring, and in the interest of group cohesion (e.g. Pam & Kemper, 1993).

On this occasion the nurse tells the patient that if his appraisal of the situation is accurate then leaving the group is, of course, the correct course of action and one which she would encourage him to take. She also suggests that, before leaving, he could hear the thoughts of others in the group on the matter. They have all been in his position. None of them was comfortable in their first meeting. Would he listen to their advice before he leaves? He reluctantly agrees and listens as the others talk of their initial discomfort and of how their views have now changed.

He opts to stay and begins to speak more specifically about the source of his discomfort. He is anxious about being observed via the one-way screen. As the words leave his mouth my own anxiety level rises as I view the proceedings from the other side of it.

I have long considered 'live' supervision to be the method *par excellence* in work with groups and families. I have also witnessed its use as a vile instrument of patient oppression by professionals, used more to define the limits of professional power than as a tool of therapy.

I have made a number of attempts to flatten the hierarchy in this regard. For example, in one inpatient unit, the patients changed places with the staff observers at the end of the meetings. Instead of meeting behind closed doors, the staff discussion of group process took place with the patients observing from behind the screen. At the end of this discussion the group and the observers met in the same room in order that the latter could respond to the comments of the former.

The idea was to democratise and demystify the process of therapy. Patients observed the staff meetings via the one-way screen, just as they had been observed by the staff. At the end of the meetings they commented on processes going on between staff members, just as the staff had commented on what had gone on in the group. They also participated in workshops on group theory to equip them with the language required. The task of conceptualisation was a shared one and the focus of discussion often involved challenges to the position adopted by staff.

The surface picture was one of patients and staff working in equal partnership, but how much of this was illusory is difficult to say with any certainty. The outcome of today's discussion is that the patients are in agreement that the discomfort caused by the one-way screen passes with time and that the screen can be useful.

Unfortunately it is difficult to discriminate between a relationship which is truly collaborative and one which is not. The combination of the 'one down' position that patients occupy, and the fact that they are desperate for assistance, is likely to inhibit them from complaining or making negative statements to the 'professionals'. My presence behind the one-way screen has often been challenged, but on only one occasion have patients asked me to leave the room, and then at the very next meeting of the group they insisted that I return.

To complicate matters further, in their appraisal of what is 'helpful', patients overestimate the contribution of therapists and can believe that they have been understood in some profound way, even when the therapist has understood little (Yalom & Elkin, 1974). Banton *et al.* (1985) commented on the tendency of patients to bestow unwarranted praise on therapists, relating this to issues of power inherent in the role of the nurse/custodian as therapist:

'This both flatters the worker's narcissism and makes for passive, easily managed clients, but it has nothing to do with helping people make sense of their own experience and much to do with further alienating them from their own capacity to think and comprehend, as well as from the inexpert but genuine responsiveness of those around them to their suffering.'

I view the 'inexpert' assistance patients have to offer each other as the core of what happens in the group. The nursing staff usually have little experience of the condition which they refer to as 'depression', for example. It is even rarer for them to have experienced hallucinations or delusions.

Although I am far from certain that what I see happening here constitutes true collaboration between patients and staff, I am convinced that patients collaborate with each other. There is little opportunity for 'flattered narcissism' on the part of the nurses here. They are more likely to hear complaints, and the credit for anything beneficial which happens is seldom given to the staff. It is customary for patients on leaving the group to speak of the benefits they have received, but it is unusual for them to attribute these benefits to the staff. Patients more often cite other patients as having made a difference in their lives during their time in the group.

I also view each group as an opportunity for learning, for myself and the other nurses involved, and agree with Peplau (1990, p. 90): 'All contacts which nurses have with patients are potential learning experiences for both parties: nurses enrich and refine their expertise, and patients expand and improve their competencies and their self knowledge.'

Both parties have much to learn. Patients come here to be cured and they view the professionals as the purveyors of the cure. They do not come with the expectation that they will cure themselves. They are often bemused by an approach which requires them to arrive at solutions to problems through their own efforts and that they 'transform themselves' (Peplau, 1994).

I am often reminded of one patient's response to this suggestion: 'I am here because I have had a nervous breakdown and I expect you to rectify the situation. I am also in need of a haircut. What would happen if my barber started handing scissors to his customers and telling them that haircuts are best arrived at by their own efforts? The result would be bad haircuts. He would soon be out of business and so will you if this is the best you have to offer.'

There are parallels here with my own relationship with the nurses, as a trainer and supervisor. This same room will be used this afternoon as the venue for the introductory groupwork course involving a dozen or so people from various mental health organisations throughout the country. The tensions involved in my role as trainer are as formidable as those faced by the nurses in this morning's group. My thoughts on training and supervision have changed considerably since the course began 10 years ago. By the beginning of the 1990s my conceptual framework was becoming broader and had encompassed a diverse range of influences.

This led to something of a crisis around the beginning of the 1990s when the expectation of course participants was driven by a culture of hi-tech hard science where everything needed to be 'sorted' quickly and cheaply. Group approaches were becoming much more popular but they had to be very precisely packaged and, if at all possible, they had to be uncontaminated by 'messy human entanglement'.

My job was perceived to be that of provider of answers to questions such as: What works? What doesn't work? Many of the participants expected that they would leave with a pristine model accompanied by a parts guarantee. Many of them were disappointed. We were moving in opposite directions – they asked for certainty, I gave only the assurance that I was absolutely certain about nothing.

Most of the staff in my own organisation preferred cognitive-behavioural interventions and neat packages of therapy whose outcome could be precisely measured within the prevailing positivistic paradigm. In order to facilitate this 'measurement', each package had to be the same. No interaction between patients was required or even desirable. A therapist with a script and an overhead projector would be much more reliable.

From a conceptual point of view, my position was that there was no one true way, and that choice of conceptual framework was irrelevant provided that the framework used had the power to liberate patients. I occasionally cited Yalom's view that, in this respect, astrology was as good a model as any. This did nothing to enhance my already diminishing popularity.

The 'Class of 95' is more open to exploration of alternative approaches. It is now more fashionable to speak of groups which involve the participation of patients. This may be due to the failure of the 'neat packages' to deliver the goods and it may be evidence of an increased willingness to live without the security which they appeared to offer.

In any event, I have fallen short of the mark of arriving at an authoritative 'version' of the role of the mental health nurse. My current belief is that such a task is not possible, given the incomprehensibility of the field and the impossible tensions and contradictions which that role involves. Perhaps this failure is no bad thing. I take comfort from Banton *et al.*'s (1985, p. 21) view that:

> 'Possession of a discourse that solves the problems of the real world in one sweep can be comforting, but it can also lead away from action by failing to note the alternative discourses that are also available, perhaps also representing part of "the truth".'

References

Banton, R., Clifford, P., Frosh, S., Lousada, J. & Rosenthall, J. (1985) *The Politics of Mental Health*. London, MacMillan.

Busfield, J. (1986) *Managing Madness: Changing Ideas and Practice*. Hutchinson, London.

Clinton, M. (1985) Training psychiatric nurses: why theory into practice won't go. In *Psychiatric Nursing* (A. Altschul ed.), Churchill Livingstone, Edinburgh, pp. 132–149.

Collister, B. (1988) Introduction: sharing perceptions. In *Psychiatric Nursing: Person to Person* (Collister B. ed.), Edward Arnold, London.

Cooper, D. (1978) *The Language of Madness*. Penguin, Harmondsworth.

Cormack, D. (1976) *Psychiatric Nursing Observed. A Descriptive Study of the Work of the Charge Nurse in Acute Admission Wards of Psychiatric Hospitals*. Royal College of Nursing, London.

Cormack, D. (1983) *Psychiatric Nursing Described*. Churchill Livingstone, Edinburgh.

John, A. (1961) *A Study of the Psychiatric Nurse*. E. & S. Livingstone, Edinburgh.

Johnstone, I. (1989) *Users and Abusers of Psychiatry: A Critical Look at Traditional Psychiatric Practice*. Routledge, London.

Kibel, H.D. (1987) Contributions of the group psychotherapist to education on the psychiatric unit: teaching through group dynamics. *International Journal of Group Psychotherapy* **37** (1), 1–29.

Laing, R.D. (1961) *The Self and Others*. Tavistock, London.

Laing, R.D. (1967) *The Politics of Experience*. Penguin, Harmondsworth.

Lego, S. (1992) Biological psychiatry and psychiatric nursing in America. *Archives of Psychiatric Nursing* **11** (3), 147–150.

Levine, H.B. (1980) Milieu biopsy: the place of group psychotherapy on the inpatient ward. *International Journal of Group Psychotherapy* **37** (1), 77–93.

Miller, P. & Rose, N. (1986) *The Power of Psychiatry*. Polity, Cambridge.

Mintz, M. (1964) *The Therapeutic Nightmare*. Houghton Mifflin, Boston.

Pam, A. & Kemper, S. (1993) The captive group: guidelines for group therapists in the inpatient setting. *International Journal of Group Psychotherapy* **43** (4), 419–438.

Peplau, H. (1952) *Interpersonal Relations in Nursing*. Putnam, New York.

Peplau, H.E. (1990) Interpersonal relations model. Principles and general applications. In *Psychiatric and Mental Health Nursing: Theory and Practice* (Reynolds, W. & Cormack, D. eds), Chapman and Hall, London.

Peplau, H.E. (1994) Psychiatric mental health nursing: challenge and change. *Journal of Psychiatric and Mental Health Nursing* **1**, 3–7.

Porter, S. (1992) The poverty of professionalism: a critical analysis of strategies for the occupational advancement of nursing. *Journal of Advanced Nursing* **17**, 720–726.

Powell, D. (1982) *Learning to Relate. A Study of Student Psychiatric Nurses' Views of their Preparation and Training*. Royal College of Nursing, London.

Reed, P.G. (1987) Constructing a conceptual framework for psychosocial nursing. *Journal of Psychosocial Nursing* **25** (2), 24–28.

Render, H. (1947) *Nurse–Patient Relationships in Psychiatry*. McGraw-Hill, New York.

Ruttan, J.S., Alonso, A. & Groves, J.E. (1988) Understanding defences in group psychotherapy. *International Journal of Group Psychotherapy* **34** (4), 449–464.

Sills, G.M. (1977) Research in the field of psychiatric nursing 1952–1977. *Nursing Research* **26** (3), 201–206.

Stone, W.N., Rodenhauser, P. & Markert, R.J. (1991) Combining group psychotherapy and pharmacotherapy. *International Journal of Group Psychotherapy* **41**, 449–464.

Szasz, T. (1963) *Law, Liberty and Psychiatry*. Macmillan, New York.

Szasz, T. (1972) *The Myth of Mental Illness*. Granada, London.

Towell, D. (1975) *Understanding Psychiatric Nursing*. Royal College of Nursing, London.

Travelbee, J. (1969) *Intervention in Psychiatric Nursing: Process in the One to One Relationship*. F.A. Davis, Philadelphia.

Wing, J.K. & Brown, G.W. (1970) *Institutionalism and Schizophrenia. A Comparative*

Study of Three Mental Hospitals, 1960–1968. Cambridge University Press, Cambridge.

Yalom, I.D. (1983) *Inpatient Group Psychotherapy.* Basic Books, New York.

Yalom, I.D. & Elkin, G. (1974) *Every Day gets a Little Bit Closer. A Twice Told Theory.* Basic Books, New York.

Zaslav, M.R. & Kalb, R.D. (1989) Medicine as metaphor and medium in group psychotherapy with psychiatric inpatients. *International Journal of Group Psychotherapy* **39** (4), 457–468.

10　The Mental Health Nurse as Rhetorician

Stephen Tilley

Introduction

In this chapter I will first recount three episodes from my practice as a mental health nurse (MHN), then use the metaphor of 'the MHN as rhetorician' as a device for investigating some ambiguities in these episodes. Metaphors can be used to illuminate something about which little is known (my practice, and the practice of MHNs more generally), by relating it to something about which more is known (rhetoric is an ancient and still viable discipline).

Episode 1 – A man running towards the window
As a student psychiatric nurse on night duty I was told to go urgently to the neighbouring ward. Walking into the ward I saw an old man running away from me towards the far end of the corridor, where a table stood next to a window. I caught up with him as he leaped onto the table, and wheeled him about and back down to the ground.

Episode 2 – A door and 'karma'
One time during my training as a psychiatric nurse, a senior nurse told me to accompany a trained nurse to a police station in a nearby town to bring in a patient under the terms of the Mental Health Act. We arrived to find several policemen standing at a door inside the station. We were told that behind the door was a young foreign man who had become disturbed and violent while staying at the nearby Buddhist centre. The police had locked him in and were debating how to proceed. It became clear that they thought it necessary to open the door and rush him, to control him while the doctor present gave him an injection. I asked if I could talk to him instead – at least try to convince him to come to hospital. They agreed, but with evident scepticism, to let me try. I stood at the door aware of the presence of the officers and nurse behind me. I called to the man. He replied in broken English and I found it difficult to understand him.

One of the words I could make out was 'karma'. I tried to relate to him on this basis, saying that his karma now was that he had to come to hospital. It could not be avoided. It would happen. We wanted him to come voluntarily. But he would have to come. It was his karma.

As we talked his voice rose, and so did the tension on my side of the door. Finally the senior police officer signalled that the time had come to move. Briefly the plan was rehearsed. The police put on their gloves. We went into the room and used force to restrain and sedate the man, and transport him to hospital.

I wondered many times thereafter what I had been trying to do – to construct by the use of the term 'karma' some basis of communication that would have allowed this person to be taken from his frame of reference to ours, without the use of force.

I was trying to establish a frame of understanding with the German behind the door, a person unseen, whose second language was my first, by use of a term I could hardly construe, not knowing fully the sense he might make of it. I was trying to move him to see that he must do something we wanted him to do. This attempt failed, another way of moving him, expressed in the language of hand, glove and chemical, conveyed the same metamessage.

Episode 3 – My friend and I

My friend came to see me and we talked. Some things my friend said unsettled me. He narrated a sequence of events around his suddenly giving up his work, due, he said, to a vague sense that things were 'not right'.

I was worried, because I could not quite follow some parts of the story my friend told. I was not sure whether that vagueness was due to some problem in my understanding, or to a problem in my friend's thinking. Some time ago my friend went through a phase where he thought that neighbours were conspiring against him, in league with others engaged in horrible practices. He ended up admitted to a mental hospital, diagnosed as 'manic'. I wondered if this was a recurrence.

But, I thought to myself, I do understand some of what he is saying. Moreover, I was flattered that he thought that I understood. His attributing understanding to me seemed to enable me to grasp more of what he said, even what might be seen as odd or 'crazy'. He said that I seemed to be able to hear and understand what he was saying, and that he was looking for someone who would understand it. He thought that I was the person. I felt this as a burden, an obligation, though I wanted also to be his friend and someone who could understand him. But to my vigilant ears even the emphasis he placed on our being friends seemed overdone, not the normal pub conversation.

For me all this raised questions about my construction of my friend as possibly mentally ill (cf. Smith's 1978 account of the role of friends in constructing someone as mentally ill). Afterwards, I found myself linking our talk to my concerns with rhetoric and persuasion – how was I persuaded or not persuaded that what he was saying made sense or indicated mental illness? I heard him as trying to persuade me that I would understand or did understand.

I heard him as arguing on the basis of an assumption of connections between things. For example, he told a story about finding a dying duck on the road the day he quit his job. He cried when the duck died in his car. He found the place to bury it, near the still point in the river – a river that he thinks is 'in him' – in right relation to four trees. He said he trusted that I would understand the depth of his feeling, his compassion for the duck; that I would accept that what he was experiencing related to compassion and to the Buddhism he practises. He trusted that I understood what he meant when he said that the river was 'in him'.

I saw my friend again some days later. He told me more about three episodes over the past few years when he had experienced changes in feelings, perceptions and mood, that had led to his being hospitalised as 'manic'. He said that he had not revealed most of this to his doctors, nor to his wife, and he told me things gradually. On those three occasions, he had started waking early in the morning, with 'visions' of various kinds (some of demons, which he also saw in rooms during these spells; some of eyes, in particular eyes opening, especially one eye which he thought of as his third eye, opening, giving him knowledge). He had a feeling of lightness, tears came to his eyes. It was a gentle change for a few days, and he experienced this phase as something positive. He had access to visions and to knowledge that he had never had before. Things were intensely meaningful, connected. But over a few days, things speeded up, he got more involved in trying to do too many things, got suspicious of others, things got in his way, he came up against things and other people. On each occasion he packed in his job. On one occasion staff from the nearest mental hospital came to take him in.

He was telling me these things, I think, as a friend, to see if I understood what he had experienced. He told, too, of his experience of profound meanings in natural things and places, stones, trees, the river. Especially stones. And especially the river. He knows stones; that they are not to be broken, that they are meant to be in particular places. He is aware that things go in threes, and has found out that three is the special number for Celts. He sees his powers and experiences as shamanic.

I am persuaded that my friend has some particular knowledge and some unusual powers. He knows these things and I trust and respect his knowledge. It is not the knowledge, the main or accepted knowledge, of our times. I told him about a book by Podvoll (1990) which recounts the phenomenology of 'madness', the experience of power, of the speeding of time, and so on. He seemed to recognise these accounts as like his experience. What he wanted to know was, did they get over it? Did they get better or recover? I realised how shaken he had been by these three episodes. (He hopes that because there have been three episodes, and three is a special number, they are over.)

But I felt as if I had failed, in the end, to connect to him and with him. There were tears in his eyes at one point before I left. He said 'I'm not mad' and looked sharply at me. I said that the term 'madness' was just one way to characterise the experience, that I thought of it in terms of his experience. But somehow I think that that hurt him. And near the end I was trying to get a sense of what he was asking me for. He said that, knowing my interests, he wondered if what he had experienced could be of use to me in my line of work, meaning interest in mental illness.

I sense that my friend does not want to be deprived of these experiences that are so meaningful, eye-opening, empowering (in a radically different sense than that in which the term is usually used – shamanic empowerment), yet awful in intensity and consequence. But he is fearful of the disruption to his life, work, relationships. And he said that most of his close relatives had had periods of mental illness; he fears how things may go. Also, I sensed that he wanted someone to acknowledge and recognise the knowledge and experience he had, not discount it or explain it away.

Standing back from experience: an excursion into rhetoric

These episodes may not be particularly representative of mental health nursing practice. Certainly, any MHN could think of her or his own practice and recount episodes which might convey different impressions of the work.

What is clear, though, is that the situations I have described are all, in different ways, problematic. Part of the problem has been that each episode is open to different interpretations – of what was going on, of my role, of the situation of the person to whom I was trying to relate. In the first episode, I came into a situation and without hesitation restrained and redirected another person. In the second, I was, on the one hand, trying to help the unfortunate man behind the door; on the other, I clearly participated in doing something to him that he did not want done. My status as actor, my acts, the scene itself – all are ambiguous and open to contradictory readings. Similarly, in the third episode, I had great difficulty understanding what my friend and I were doing in our interaction; what his actions and words meant to me, and *vice versa*.

The problematic qualities of the episodes increase with the distance from the hospital. An action of 'corralling' an elderly man seemed unremarkable in the context of an admission ward; while my uncertainty about role and relationship, based on my being positioned in relation to competing definitions of the situation and of what was required of me, was magnified in the unfamiliar setting of the police station, and magnified again in sitting with my friend in a pub. Ambiguities are more evident when nursing is de-centred from its traditional seat of power and knowledge, the hospital.

The way that I have tried to make sense of these ambiguities is to look at them from the perspective of rhetoric. Rhetoric is a field of knowledge about how to accomplish understanding and remedy misunderstanding (Stanton & Schwartz, 1954; Burke, 1969a, 1969b), and how to persuade another, or indeed oneself, that a particular view or line of action is appropriate. Insofar as the particular problems posed by these episodes have the same general counterpart – how can disputes and ambiguities be resolved? – the metaphor of 'the nurse as rhetorician' becomes relevant.

Logoi, ethos and pathos

There is a long tradition of thinking about rhetoric and the means of persuasion. Persuasion was seen, classically, to depend on three elements: '[Aristotle argued] that persuasion depends on the oratorical act as a whole – not merely on the proofs, or *logoi*, in the speech itself, but also on the manner, or *ethos*, of the rhetor and on the emotional response, or *pathos*, evoked in the auditors.' (Mooney, 1994, p 31). Frank and Frank (1991, p. 68), in their analysis of the rhetorical dimension of psychotherapy, likewise draw on Aristotle's view that: ' … the rhetorician seeks to influence hearers by (1) evincing a personal character or *ethos* that will win the confidence of the listener; (2) engaging the listener's emotions; and (3) providing a truth, real or apparent, by argument'. This tripartite analysis will be drawn on throughout the rest of the chapter.

Logoi

Proofs, arguments, truth – all presuppose knowledge. What *kind* of knowledge does the rhetorician have? Some routes to persuasion, such as logic or mathematical proof, give a degree of certainty; via others, for example interpretation of texts, such certainty is less likely, and indeed a less specific accord may be the aim. Mooney (1994, p. 31) outlines Aristotle's sense of oratory (rhetoric) as:

> 'a logic of persuasion or argumentation … the kind of reasoning that goes on among nonspecialists in matters that are merely or mainly probable.'

What is necessary, then, is a set of adequate distinctions between kinds of human activity. Mooney (1994, p. 5) presents Aristotle's analysis of art, prudence, dialectic, and rhetoric:

> 'Certain activities, such as baking bread or cobbling shoes, might rely on "art" (*techné*) – practical knowledge culled from repeated experience. For the rest, however, mortals must depend on mere prudence (*phronésis*) – a facility acquired through studied circumspection. Not all men, however, are prudent, he realized, and even those who are will disagree in deliberating courses of action. Besides being prudent, consequently, men must also argue, seeking to make plausible the actions they favor by relating them to commonly held assumptions. Such everyday discourse, not limited to specialists or to certain subjects of inquiry, Aristotle called dialectic. Enriched by charm and appeals to emotion and adapted to instances of formal oratory, dialectic in turn becomes rhetoric, that form of public reasoning "in such matters as we deliberate upon without arts or systems to guide us, in the hearing of persons who cannot take in at a glance a complicated argument."'

Nor is persuasion necessarily consciously intended. '[rhetoric] lies midway between aimless utterance and speech directly purposive' (Burke, 1969b, p. xiii). Aristotle's highlighting of the 'everyday' quality of dialectic discourse has a counterpart in the central role that common sense plays in rhetoric. Yet even common sense has an ethical dimension, conveyed by the notion of 'prudence'. Mooney (1994, p. 37) cites Cicero's view that:

'The wisdom required of the orator was not the theoretical science or nature or the subtle discipline of logic ... but the study of human life, of men and morals, what the ancients call prudence and the Stoics ethics or moral philosophy ... These were intrinsically public sciences, disciplines of the forum, the court, the marketplace ...'

Similarly, Frank and Frank (1991, p. 66) argue that 'psychotherapy may be more closely akin to rhetoric than to applied behavioural science':

'The truths of science, which deals with controllable, repeatable, objective phenomena, are empirically demonstrable. The truths of both rhetoric and psychotherapy, however, are far less certain. Dialectics, a form of disciplined conversation, seeks to approach rhetorical truths.'

Ethos
It may be assumed here that 'disciplined' connotes a sense of talk and action regulated primarily by the intention to avoid misunderstanding, and to reach shared views. Likewise, 'conversation' suggests talking that is not merely directed towards knowledge. One of the main means of persuasion, of establishing shared conviction, is identification (Burke, 1969b). Identification can facilitate cooperation, for example getting the nurse alongside the patient, or the patient alongside the nurse, so that cooperation toward some goal is facilitated. Identification can be accomplished by relating arguments to the basic elements of common sense, shared by speaker and audience. The classical rhetorician learned to relate specific arguments to 'common places' or 'common topics', on which different stances could be taken, different positions established. One way to move the audience to see one's point of view is to find some common ground, and one way of doing that is to orientate in terms of a common place or *topic*. This is essentially a matter of focusing attention (see Lipson & Lipson, 1996).

Mooney (1994, p. 33) argues that:

'... no claimant to rhetorical art, however routine his duties or leaden his ways, could fail to pursue what is, in every account, the aim and end of all oratory: to so marshal *res* and *verba*, thoughts and words, ideas and language, as to say what is -, at the moment - "called for," suited to the occasion, fitting and proper, appropriate and decorous, and so advance the cause of public life.'

Pathos
The aim, in effect, is to answer the question: 'What is to be done?'. This question has practical and ethical dimensions.

The means and elements of rhetoric have been sketched, but what of aims? Practically, a distinction was made in classical rhetoric between forensic rhetoric, aimed at producing shared understanding of 'Who's to blame, where did this come from?' and deliberative rhetoric, aimed at producing shared understanding of 'What are we going to do about this?'. I will suggest below that these are counterparts to nursing assessment ('Why is the patient here now?') and implementation of care ('What do we have to do for her?'). Forensic rhetoric leaves open the question of whether blame will be sought in biological 'causes', faults in personality, or lack of will, for example. Deliberative rhetoric is the sphere of reasoning about appropriate responses, given these senses of what to 'blame'.

According to classical literature, rhetorical skills could be used in the service of the speaker's own interests, or those of (or those shared with) his audience:

> 'As the base rhetorician uses language to increase his own power, to produce converts to his own cause, and to create loyal followers to his own person, so the noble rhetorician uses language to wean men from their inclination to depend on authority, to encourage them to think and speak clearly, and to teach them to be their own masters . . .'

> 'Rhetoric at its truest sense (that is, noble rhetoric) seeks to perfect men by showing them better versions of themselves . . .'
>
> (Weaver, cited in Szasz, 1979, p. 20)

The practical and the ethical are thus intertwined:

> 'By discussing only one side of an issue, by mentioning cause without consequence or consequence without cause, acts without agents or agents without agency, [the base rhetorician] often successfully blocks definition and cause-and-effect reasoning.'
>
> (Weaver, cited in Szasz, 1979, p. 20)

Return to experience: versions of karma

The reader may have been struck by the contrast between the narration of episodes of practice which opened this chapter, and the subsequent abstract, rational exposition of rhetoric. Noting this contrast, the reader might think that the metaphor of rhetorician cannot accommodate the practice of mental health nursing. Certainly, I did not think of myself, wittingly, as a rhetorician or persuader during much of the time I practised as a nurse. The 'proof' of connection between MHNs and rhetoricians may be suspect.

However, the reader will note the emphasis, in the definition of rhetoric, on ethos and pathos as well as on logoi. Precisely because the episodes are ambiguous, open to different interpretations, attention is drawn to issues of ethos and pathos, the character of the speaker and the impact on the audience. I will therefore now review the second and third episodes to indicate that the metaphor can be useful in shaping understandings of practice.

I will focus particularly on use, and misuse, of the term 'karma' in episodes 2 and 3, relating this to the idea of the 'base rhetorician' and the 'good rhetorician' (Weaver, cited in Szasz, 1979). In retrospect I think that I misused the term in the 'door' episode. Not only did I not understand its meaning; my use of the term in that context was coercive, an example of base rhetoric. I was trying to use the term 'karma' to get the person behind the door to comply with what the police, the psychiatric institution, the doctor present, wanted him to do. I did it without any consideration of the implications of the term for the 'audience' (both the man behind the door, and those with me on the other side, of the door and of the issue). Talking to the man about 'your karma' and saying that 'you have to come in', I diverted attention from the real agents and act. I felt like someone misusing a connection (possible counter-cultural affinities) to do coercive work on behalf of others (the psychiatrists, general practitioner and police). I felt shame.

Why should I have felt shame? This depends on what shame is, and the conditions under which one experiences it. Bedford (1986, p. 21) claims that:

> 'In general, it is true to say of someone 'He is ashamed of so-and-so' only if what is referred to is something that he can be criticised for (the criticism is commonly, though not perhaps necessarily, moral). It is, in other words, a necessary condition for the truth of the statement that he should be at fault.'

In acknowledging shame, I am in effect identifying myself as an agent responsible for my actions in that situation; hence accountable, and liable to criticism for fault. I will return below to further consideration of the central importance of 'agency' in construction of the mental health nurse as rhetorician. I use these terms drawing on Burke's (1969a, p. xv) analysis of the 'dramatist pentad' at the heart of accounts of motivated action:

> '... any complete statement about motives will offer some kind of answers to these five questions: what was done (act), when or where it was done (scene), who did it (agent), how he did it (agency), and why (purpose).'

Implicit in this analysis is the sense that an 'agent' is responsible for the act. An 'agency' is the means used by the agent to do the act. Colonel Mustard (agent) with the hammer (agency) in the billiard room (scene) did the murder (act): but why (purpose)?

The examples I have given indicate that persuasion and interpretation may be acutely problematic matters. In episode 2, the door is a metaphor for the barriers that stand between two sides of an argument. The rhetorical tradition emphasises the importance of ethos and pathos, as well as logos. I felt after episode 2 that I could not trust myself, nor could the German trust me. I had acted in good faith to avert a worse course of action, but had failed to do so. I had tried to move, as it were, through the door to be alongside the man, to exert pathos, but had instead acted as a base rhetorician.

I have recast the meaning of episode 2, long after the event, by making connections between subjects which I did not set out to relate to each other. Now, through the conversations with my friend recounted in episode 3, I have the opportunity to revisit some of the issues involved. I have returned to the question of how to respond to the possibility of there being (of seeing and making) connections between events, and to the interpretation of experience linked to an alternative system of belief (karma or shamanic power). Indeed, after seeing my friend, I asked myself whether he was giving me an opportunity to solve a problem of particular significance to me. When I thought further, I realised this problem reached back deep into my childhood, about the ways that I formulated my sense of who I am and what I am in the world to do: the problem of how to respond to, and care for, another whose acts and thinking place him or her outwith the bounds of common experience and understanding. I sense that my friend may be a noble rhetorician, indirectly showing me a possible 'better version' of myself as an MHN. He has somehow returned me to the topic of karma, the return itself.

Learning based on this kind of experience and reflection is long-term, open in structure, based on development of a matrix of personal concerns related to wider issues in literature and in subsequent interaction. My learning about mental health nursing and its meanings has sometimes been learning by indirection or 'perambulation' (C.S. Peirce's term), not deliberate. I have learned by committing myself to positions in arguments and then following the implications for self and others. Such learning may indeed be karmic.

The MHN as rhetorician

The above account of rhetoric can be related not only to the particulars of specific situations, but also to general topics in mental health nursing. In this section, I will explore this issue in terms of logoi, ethos and pathos: the kind(s) of knowledge MHNs use, MHNs' character, and the effects they seek to produce in others.

Firstly, rhetoric is relevant to mental health nursing specifically and crucially with respect to issues of knowledge. There is a body of literature that sees MHNs are 'non-specialists' in the sense that their body of knowledge relates to things that lay people know about (cf. Robinson, 1985, regarding health visitors' knowledge). That this is the case is considered problematic; indeed, the lack of a specialist expertise has been seen as a fundamental problem for mental health nurses, posing for them problems of legitimacy in face-to-face interaction as well as in the sphere of professionalisation (May & Kelly, 1982) Thus, given the lack of consensus on the appropriate paradigm for mental health nursing, claims in this field *must* be about what is probable and arguable, in contrast to the scientific ideal of knowledge which is certain and demonstrable.

In the face of discord among theoreticians, no authoritative, legislative single view can dominate. Moreover, as the 'problems' which lead to people being seen as 'mentally ill' may be diverse and not easily categorisable, consisting of 'residual' violations of the social order of everyday life (cf. Scheff, 1966), and as the aim of work with the people having such problems is to restore them to the 'paramount reality' of everyday life (cf. Tilley, 1995a, on Berger & Luckmann's metaphor of therapy as recovery of 'strays' from the 'paramount reality'), such work must be based on experience and directed towards what is feasible in the local setting rather than 'correct' in any decontextualised or theoretical sense. Indeed, common sense, rather than being a hindrance to nurses in their quest for theoretical knowledge, can legitimately be regarded as the essential form of knowledge for mental health nursing practice.

The centrality of common sense to mental health nursing practice is one of the main grounds for asserting the relevance of the metaphor of mental health nurse as rhetorician. In the rhetorical tradition, knowledge was constructed through argument based on the 'common places' or *topoi*. Among the common places of psychiatric and mental health nursing practice, the main topic is 'illness' itself. In settings where the medical or psychiatric model dominates the ethos, answering the question 'Why is this patient here, now?' entails focusing on the topic of illness. The model does rhetorical work. The centrality of 'illness' as a common place has been challenged in critiques of the 'medical model', where the topic is shifted from 'illness' to 'rights'. Szasz is a master of this shift of topic, and some discourses of the current users' movement likewise focus on rights. However, psychiatrists and some MHNs work to move the topic back to illness, in order to lead nurses to care of the 'most ill' (Wooff & Goldberg, 1988; Gournay, 1995) or onto the topic of the 'dangerousness' of 'mentally ill' people (highlighting recent headline-making cases).

Common places have to be established and maintained. This is always rhetorical work. The other in an argument might try to move one off the topic. For example, in arguments over community care for the mentally ill, one might want to resist moving onto the topic of 'dangerousness' of psychiatric patients (even if one is able to assert, citing statistics, that the mentally ill are not more dangerous), and try instead to move onto a preferred topic (the right to live in a place of one's own choosing) (see Cowan, 1997).

The link between this metaphoric sense of 'moving' others, and the literal sense, should be highlighted. Persons' rights and obligations regarding removal to a mental hospital under 'sections' of the Mental Health Act 1983 (England and Wales) or the Mental Health Act 1984 (Scotland), or to treatment in the community under a Compulsory Treatment Order (Mental Health (Patients in the Community) Act 1995), are topics made relevant by people in real arguments. The 'move' of patients, first into asylums and hospitals, now into the community, is mediated by discourses constructed rhetorically to make illness or rights the topic of argument (cf. Cowan, 1994).

A second aspect of knowledge and rhetoric relevant to MHNs is the distinction between deliberative rhetoric ('What are we going to do about this?') and forensic rhetoric ('Who's to blame, where did this come from?'). This distinction is clearly to be seen in two cognate questions around which nurses in psychiatric admission wards were found to organise their practice (Tilley, 1995a): 'Why is she (the patient) here now?' is the counterpart to forensic rhetoric; and 'What do we have to do for her?' is the counterpart to deliberative rhetoric. Forensic rhetoric concerns the making of cases through attribution of causes. This is what MHNs do when they apply some 'model' – behavioural, psychodynamic, nursing – to a patient's 'presentation'. They do so in order to set the stage for deliberation on what to do with or for the patient.

Clearly then, the rhetorical tradition casts light on current reasoning about psychiatric nursing. Vico thought that 'When men act publicly, or when they urge a course of action upon others, they must be ready with their reasons' (Mooney, 1994, p. 4). Hence, nurses as self-aware rhetoricians must be 'ready with their reasons'.

Current nursing discourses on knowledge depend on claims being made or disputed on the basis of evidence. Some of the current debates in nursing journals about the *appropriate* focus for MHNs (Gournay, 1995; Brooker *et al.*, 1996) can be construed in terms of the call for evidence-based practice, and the attempt to establish a valid, reliable basis for practice development. Others have more to do with establishing the legitimacy of topics, for example 'caring' in mental health nursing (Barker *et al.*, 1995). These attempts to determine the appropriate focus of work of MHNs entail issues of morality (what is proper, right) and power (what are the effects of MHNs practices; who is to direct them?). For example, Barker (1991), chastising those nurses whom he regards as having come to see themselves as 'angels' able to 'rise above' emotionality and common humanity, as *other* than those they care for, tries to mobilise nurses to follow the proper 'path' (Barker, 1991).

Only some of these current nursing discourses are recognisably 'scientific'. The claim that the MHN is a scientist, or ought to be one, is itself subject to rhetorical dispute. The 'MHN as scientist' is but one, limited, representation of the MHN as someone committed to knowing or understanding self and others. In characterising the MHN as rhetorician one opens the prospect of the MHN committed to 'the study of human life'. The knowledge base will be a 'public science', a 'discipline' of the public place. This connotes the MHN in the public places of day rooms of admission wards and long stay wards in hospitals, and in the community, seeking prudence and reason rather than 'scientific' truth. (The tension between 'scientific' and 'dialectic' conceptions of the MHN's work had a counterpart in current debates in psychology. In response to a reductionist scientific account, Billig (1987) represents mind as argument, and thinking as essentially dilemmatic and rhetorical.)

Recalling now Aristotle's tripartite analysis of knowledge – theoretical science, art and prudence – we can say that recent nursing literature emphasises only two of these, theory and art. Prudence has been relatively neglected, though matters related to prudence underlie some research-based interpretations of nursing. Prudence can be thought of as conduct which carefully avoids undesired consequences (*The Concise Oxford Dictionary*, 1976). In the human realm, undesired consequences are not decontextualised; instead, they follow from action based on the ways of that part of the world, and are the work of actors in that part of the world.

In a main strand of literature in psychiatric nursing (Altschul, 1972; Diers & Leonard, 1966) researchers noted nurses' failure to give accounts demonstrating 'deliberate' thinking in their interaction with patients. The nurses in Altschul's study claimed to work on the basis of 'common sense' even when the theoretical base to their work was not evident to the researcher (Altschul, 1972) – the logoi were not clearly convincing, at least to Altschul. She called into question the legitimacy of the claim of 'common sense' on the grounds that different nurses interpreted or responded to the same situation in different ways, and adopted 'contradictory' approaches to patients (Altschul, 1972, pp. 146–150). She saw their 'intuitive approach' as 'wasteful of therapeutic opportunities' (Altschul, 1972, p. 194), and the 'theoretical basis' of psychiatric nursing practice was not evident (Altschul, 1972, p. 196). The nurses seemed to fall back on a claim that the researcher *should* understand, that anyone would do it the way the nurses did.

In a context in which the nurse can be seen as accountable to the researcher, and indirectly to the audience of the research (readers, students), these nurses can be seen as imprudent, in that they did not give accounts of the sort that would allow them to avoid the undesired consequence of their work being regarded as improper, insofar as it was not deliberate and rational. On the other hand, in the setting in which the nurses worked, their accounts based on reference to 'common sense' did not entail undesired consequences. More importantly, the patients to whom the nurses had to account, in the interactions on which the nurses' accounts to Altschul were based, were judged prudent or imprudent by the nurses. The nurses' interaction with the patients, their use of language in interaction, thus could be seen as prudent, or conducive to prudence on the patients' parts.

What matters, in the end, is the realm in which the undesirable consequences are to be generated. Prudence, for nurses and patients, is often construed in settings in which the nurses have greater power to create the consequences for patients. Equally, in the realm of discourses in nursing texts, nurses are subject to the consequences generated by nursing researchers (see Tilley, 1995b).

Ethos and pathos in mental health nursing

Up to this point the main emphasis in this account of the MHN as rhetorician has been on issues of knowledge. This is perhaps appropriate, given the weight attached to 'evidence-based practice', and to the pursuit of a body of knowledge to promote professionalisation. Nonetheless, there is a strand of mental health nursing literature interpretable, from a rhetorical perspective, in terms of ethos and pathos. The links between logos, ethos and pathos can be seen in a brief review of some representations of nursing practice, including what might loosely be called 'models, 'traditions', or 'versions' of that practice.

In some traditions in mental health nursing the patient was regarded as a person amenable to and worthy of persuasion. *The Handbook for Attendants on the Insane* (Medico-Psychological Association, 1919), precursor to the *Handbook for Mental Health Nurses*, is rich in advice to the MHN on the importance of persuasion. The attendant was instructed in the logoi supporting the asylum. A central platform was the attendant's role in maintaining the definition of the patient as ill:

'More important still is the fact that under no circumstances should an attendant agree for a moment with a patient's claim that he "is all right, and has nothing the matter with him" ... If it is not necessary to say anything, silence may be the best line to take; otherwise the fact that illness exists must be maintained. Improvement is often found to commence when the patient recognizes that he is out of health, and thus begins to help himself in the work of restoration.'

(Medico-Psychological Association, 1919, p. 320)

There was a major strand of explicit instruction in pathos and ethos:

'The patient is characterised thus: "In almost every case an insane person is an intensely selfish man ... self is his only study."'

(Medico-Psychological Association, 1919, p. 337)

'On taking charge of [the patient], the attendant should at once try to obtain his confidence by kindness and sympathy of manner, by watching over his comfort, and by explaining the misapprehensions which so commonly exist in the minds of the insane. In this way his ideas and feelings, the character of his delusions, and the probable nature of his conduct, may be learned. The attendant will then be better able to guide and control him in a suitable manner.'

(Medico-Psychological Association, 1919, p. 336)

Later, 'progressive' mental health nursing was linked to new drug treatments (the phenothiazines) introduced in the 1950s, which – so the story goes, made it possible for patients to respond to other kinds of treatment including those based on interaction with nurses.

In the case of the Altschul (1972) study, the persuasive powers of the nurses' arguments could be seen as depending on pathos and ethos: on a claim that the researcher is *like* them, grounded in a common sense. *Logos*, *ethos* and *pathos* are, it can now be seen, intimately connected in practical circumstances such as those that mental health nurses and patients co-construct. Appearing to make sense has a moral dimension, both in constituting one as rational and therefore entitled to respect as a certain kind of person, and in providing the basis for joint action.

It is not only people who seek to persuade. In general, current 'models' of mental health and illness can be construed as attempts to persuade the nurse and/or patient about: (1) the nature of the illness or problem; and (2) what to do to overcome or adjust to the illness or problem. Here, a very important issue related to the agency of the nurse has to be confronted. The facilities of rhetoric (whether student nurses ready to wheel old men away from dangers, arguments through the doors of locked rooms, or attentive exchanges of talk) are not the products of individual nurses. They are cultural products which individuals can pick up and use, perhaps in individual-specific ways. These facilities themselves have some measure of persuasive power. Arguments drawing on the products of theological discourse, for example, might have little persuasive force in contemporary situations of mental health care, but might have had in the past. Similarly, arguments conjuring up scientific explanations for human behaviour might now have considerable force. The nurse adopting one or other such discourse can be seen as an agency of the discourse, enacting its 'truth effects'.

Thus, a rhetorical dimension can be said to underlie, or underwrite, all 'models' of and in mental health nursing. A medical model persuades the patient to adopt a view of her or his problem as really an 'illness', and thus to comply with 'treatment'. A behavioural model persuades the patient to a view of the behavioural and cognitive antecedents and consequences of behaviour, to be courageous in confronting fears and challenging dysfunctional thinking.

I realise on reflection that a rhetorical perspective implicitly underpinned a post-registration course I did in the 1980s. As a trainee nurse behaviour therapist, I was, in effect, 'trained' as a rhetorician. We were taught how to win confidence, e.g. by using the phrase 'we know ...', to heighten conviction by taking on the mantle of authority of the specialist centre we worked in. We were taught *not* to display our ignorance, as doing so would weaken the patient's confidence in us. We were taught to engage the listener's emotions: for example, asking patients to think about a problematic issue and experience a rise or fall in anxiety, to get a sense of the problem or to demonstrate a treatment effect. And last, we provided 'a truth, real or apparent, by argument', getting the patient to recount the attempts he or she had made to manage a phobia by avoidance, then arguing (citing research) that avoidance maintained the problem and that exposure could help overcome it.

Each 'model' is supported by a wider apparatus of persuasion, now very concrete, now totally abstract. The very existence of mental hospitals persuades the wider public of the existence of mental 'illness' and the prospect of 'treatment'. Drug advertisements persuade the viewer or reader of the efficacy of a drug, in the context of acceptance of a medical model. Models are as effective as they are because they model not just knowledge or arguments based on proven facts, but also the situation in which this knowledge is considered to have 'truth effects', and the feelings towards other actors appropriate in the situations envisaged by the model. Thus, again, models are effective with respect to logoi, ethos and pathos.

Adopting a rhetorical perspective can also usefully inform reading of descriptive and prescriptive mental health nursing research, in terms of ethos and pathos. According to Shanley (1988), patients and charge nurses agree on the personal qualities they value in MHNs (ethos); the literature on 'expressed emotion' may have further implications, e.g. on the value of MHNs displaying a non-hostile and non-critical style in communication (ethos and pathos) (cf. literature on 'expressed emotion', Brooker, 1990a, 1990b).

Equally, some current practices and rationales advocated for use by MHNs are interpretable in terms of rhetoric. Two of the best-described, best-validated, most-promoted approaches to mental health care – cognitive behavioural therapy for depression and other disorders (Blackburn, 1987) and psychosocial interventions for schizophrenia (Brooker *et al.*, 1994) – clearly establish the role of argument, persuasion and/or correction of invalid thinking in mental health care. Frank and Frank (1991, p. 44) summarise the 'shared components of psychotherapies that combat demoralisation ... [and] arous[e] the patient emotionally'. Beck (1976) describes the role of the therapist in cognitive behavioural therapy. Through Socratic dialogue, the therapist helps the client to recognise flawed arguments with which the client may tyrannise himself or herself. The patient learns to challenge misconceptions, using more realistic arguments, to argue with herself or himself, monitoring the consequences for mood and behaviour of changes in thinking. In family behavioural therapy (Falloon *et al.*, 1985), a family's methods of arguing and resolving problems or disputes are related to outcomes for a family member with schizophrenia. Families are taught to reduce hostility and criticism in resolving disagreements, i.e. both to see better versions of each other and to show better versions of themselves.

The obligations of the MHN as rhetorician: agent, agency and power

The discussion to this point has indicated some ways in which rhetoric may be relevant to MHNs' practice. The account has been, to some extent, working in two directions at once. At times, MHNs have been regarded *as if they were* rhetoricians, whether or not aware of this, and perhaps despite themselves. At other times, it has been suggested that MHNs might *become* more conscious, reflexive rhetoricians, aiming at the status of the noble rhetorician. In the latter case, rhetoric is a moral art playing its part in the moral development of the nurse. This duality has a counterpart to the more general double function of metaphors in interpretation of social life. Harré (1993, p. 146) suggests that models (the example is Burke's concepts of 'dramatism'):

'are analytical tools for the description of complex social phenomena, and they are discursive tools for the accounting procedures by which actors can render their actions intelligible and warrantable.'

Metaphors can function as 'analytic models' (Harré & Secord, 1972); Goffman's (1971) dramaturgical metaphor can enable an analysis of front-stage and back-stage activities, for example. They also function as 'source models' (Harré & Secord, 1972), indicating how social interaction arises; Goffman suggests that people enact somewhat standard 'scripts' of social life. As an analytical model, the metaphor of the MHN as rhetorician enables one to *see* aspects of knowledge, power and moral order (Tilley, 1995a) – logoi, ethos and pathos – in mental health nursing practice. As a source model, the metaphor indicates that MHNs may learn through processes of persuasion, in practice and in education.

This discussion of MHN education and research accords, then, with a common-sense view that nurses, along with others in institutions, do try to persuade patients to adopt a particular view of themselves and their problems. It would be mistaken, however, to think that there is a clear consensus on what that view is. Not only are there different theoretical

perspectives, as suggested above. Equally importantly, the issue of identification, which is crucial in rhetorical work, is disputed in current discourses. On the one hand, some discourses construct the patient as the
'same' as the nurse. To get alongside the audience, it is helpful to see them
as like oneself, as sharing certain qualities, experiences, knowledge and
interests; current discourses on patients' rights, and on empowerment, are
examples (Glenister & Tilley, 1996).

On the other hand, there are discourses in which the patient is constructed as 'different' (see the excerpts, above, from the *Handbook for
Attendants on the Insane*; cf. Goffman's (1961) analysis of the mental hospital
as a 'total institution' based on 'staging of differences' between inmates and
staff). To make the matter yet more complex, some current discourses
construe the patient or client as both like the nurse and like other people
generally, in their very difference (Walsh, this volume). Anthony (1991)
and Barker (1991) presented, respectively, a nurse-become-patient's and a
nurse's view on the problems of difference posed when a nurse becomes a
patient, Barker (1991) calling on nurses to recognise the 'fact' that they are
'more alike than different'.

Patients can also be construed as rhetoricians, and thus as like MHNs.
The following excerpts suggest that persuasion is not one-sidedly the
preserve of the therapist or nurse, but is also a central aspect, for example,
of the thinking and behaviour of the person suffering depression. For
example, Wolpert (1995) wrote:

> 'There is nothing to be ashamed of if one is depressed. Depression is a serious
> illness and one should treat with contempt anyone who would argue that it is
> not, but merely, as some would claim, a mood disorder ...'

> 'I was, I believe, not so much depressed as excessively anxious – they unper-
> suasively claimed that they were really very similar – and had repeated panic
> attacks. I convinced myself with an inescapable private logic that my arrhythmia
> was uncontrollable and that I had Parkinson's disease. I developed a noticeable
> tremor. It was essential that I convince everyone of the hopelessness of my case
> and was acutely irritated that they would not agree with me.'

Clearly, arguments about the nurse being like or different from the
patient – of the utmost importance given the importance of common
sense – are tied to issues of power. Construing the MHN as a rhetorician,
in order to then equip the nurse to enhance her or his powers of persuasion, might be seen as a reinforcing of the unequal power relationship
between nurse and patient or client. Behind the arguments of individual
nurses stands the weight of potent discourses, professional status (implying expertise and benevolence), and the psychiatric institution or mental
health service. The patient's or client's arguments are not supported in a
like way. How is the MHN to act as a good rhetorician in this context?
Drawing attention to the MHN's 'power of persuasion' is likely to be
controversial in an era in which the social control function of psychiatry
is challenged and advocacy for patients is promoted. It is also likely to
collide with ideologies promoting user-led and consumer-led services.

Nonetheless, the intimate connection between issues of agenthood, agency, and power has to be addressed.

The question of agency is crucial in construing the problem of the mental health nurse as good rhetorician. This issue relates in part to the status of the patient as agent (is the patient really 'ill', and therefore not responsible, or not ill, but responsible for work on 'problems'?), and in part to the status of the MHN and to their socially-devolved powers. In their practice and in their representations of practice in accounts, MHNs have to account for themselves as moral agents (responsible for initiating and determining outcomes of their actions) and/or as non-moral, instrumental agencies, e.g. of the state or of doctors (the means by which doctors act on patients). From the interpretive point of view, adopting the rhetorical perspective helps one see the MHN's role in accounting for self as an agent or agency. From the point of view of moral art, MHNs are called 'to teach men' (and themselves) 'to be their own masters …'.

It is precisely because these issues are not obviously determined that rhetoric is an essential facility in mental health nursing. The facility is Janus-faced: on the one hand, the ability to argue about what cause and effect, agent and agency are, is both a mark of moral development and the means of moral development; equally, the MHN required to do good and to give a good account of what is done, will need rhetorical skills. The skills of rhetoric are one kind of agency which the MHN has to hand in doing her or his work. Indeed, facilities in mental health nursing more generally – from the locked side room to the group therapy room – can be regarded as essentially rhetorical.

MHNs who give accounts of finding and doing what is right at the time (Tilley 1995a), what has to be done *now*, i.e. in this situation, are practitioners 'of one of the many arts required to sustain social and political life' (Mooney, 1994, p. 36). Their arguments are always addressed to, and made appropriate for, particular audiences. For MHNs the target audiences include managers of services, interested in demonstrating 'health gain' for a population, and patients with whom the MHN might discourse on the common subjects of everyday life? In current argumentative contexts MHNs, like other nurses, have to argue for resources, and to respond in some way to the pushes and pulls of policy (e.g. to focus on work with the severely mentally ill or on others). In the professional context, the MHN is subject to discipline as a nurse required to act as an accountable practitioner (Tilley, 1995b). Increasingly, the MHN's arguments may be linked to contexts of legal accountability, or to quasi-legal processes of judgement such as standard setting and quality assurance. The MHN must be prepared to argue the case for her or his actions in courts of law, to bodies of academic or professional peers, to the client or relative, or to the person in the street.

As rhetoricians, MHNs can emphasise one pole or another of the agent–agency link. For example, the MHN acting in line with legislation (the Mental Health Act and more recent directives, e.g. on supervised discharge, may emphasise her or his role as agency (Rogers, 1996). The MHN wanting to define and protect her or his role in relation to the patient or client may emphasise agenthood. Patients or clients (the choice of terms is also a rhetorical *topos*) in interaction with MHNs and others likewise have to argue about their status as agents or agencies.

The episodes with which I began this chapter raised, so I argued, the issue of interpretation, of the problems of understanding and mis-understanding. What I think I have learned from such episodes is that the MHN has a responsibility to realise, in the situation of interaction, the conditions for action as a good or noble rhetorician and not to accept being a polemicist. In particular, the nurse has an obligation to assure his or her willingness to listen, to hear, to understand, and to do what is 'called for', taking account of the patient's or client's arguments. He or she has an obligation, based on logical, ethical and pathetic grounds, to accord the patient or client respect as a person with rights in an argument. Since 'persuasion depends on the oratorical act as a whole, not merely on the proofs, or logoi, in the speech itself, but also on the manner, or ethos, or the rhetor, and on the emotional response, or pathos, evoked in the auditors' (Mooney, 1994, p. 31), the nurse is obliged to accommodate to the ethos or manner of the (patient or client as) rhetor, and to take particular respon-sibility for her or his own pathos.

While the work of the mental health nurse must be rooted in the *sensus communis* of everyday life, in ordinary, everyday argument and discussion, the nurse has an extra ordinary obligation to address or redress unequal power relations in face-to-face interaction with patients or clients. The mental health nurse as good rhetorician will act reflexively, recognising her or his role in promulgating or resisting the current discourses of mental illness and mental health.

References

Altschul, A. (1972) *Patient–Nurse Interaction*. Churchill Livingstone, Edinburgh.

Anthony, A. (1991) Mirror images. *Nursing Times* **87** (2), 34–36.

Barker, P. (1991) Finding common ground. *Nursing Times* **87** (2), 37–38.

Barker, P.H., Reynolds, W. & Ward, T. (1995) The proper focus of nursing: a critique of the 'caring' ideology. *International Journal of Nursing Studies* **32** (4), 386–397.

Beck, A.T. (1976) *Cognitive Therapy and the Emotional Disorders*. Penguin, Har-mondsworth.

Bedford, E. (1986) Emotions and statements about them. In *The Social Construction of Emotions* (R. Harre ed.). Blackwell Publishers, Oxford.

Billig, M. (1987) *Arguing and Thinking: A Rhetorical Approach to Social Psychology*. Cambridge University Press, Cambridge.

Blackburn, I.M. (1987) *Coping with Depression*. Chambers, Edinburgh.

Brooker, C. (1990a) Expressed emotion and psychosocial intervention – a review. *International Journal of Nursing Studies* **27** (3), 267–276.

Brooker, C. (1990b) The application of the concept of expressed emotion to the role of the community psychiatric nurse – a research study, *International Journal of Nursing Studies* **27** (3), 277–285.

Brooker, C., Falloon, I. & Butterworth, A. *et al.* (1994) The outcome of training community psychiatric nurses to deliver psychosocial intervention. *British Journal of Psychiatry* **165**, 222–230.

Brooker, C., Repper, J. & Booth, A. (1996) Examining the effectiveness of community mental health nursing. *Mental Health Nursing* **16** (3), 12–15.

Burke, K. (1969a) *A Grammar of Motives*. University of California Press, Berkeley.

Burke, K. (1969b) *A Rhetoric of Motives*. University of California Press, Berkeley.

The Concise Oxford Dictionary, 6th edn. (1976) Oxford University Press, Oxford.

Cowan, S. (1994) Community attitudes towards people with mental health problems: a discourse analytic approach. *Journal of Psychiatric and Mental Health Nursing* **1** (1), 15–22.

Cowan, S.J. (1997) *Views on community care for people with mental health problems*. PhD thesis, submitted, The University of Edinburgh.

Diers, D. & Leonard, R.C. (1966) Interaction analysis in nursing research. *Nursing Research* **15** (3), 225–228.

Falloon, I., Boyd, J.L., McGill, C.W. *et al.* (1985) Family management in the prevention of morbidity of schizophrenia: clinical outcome of a 2-year longitudinal study. *Archives of General Psychiatry* **42** (9), 887–896.

Frank, J.D. & Frank, J.B. (1991) *Persuasion and Healing: A Comparative Study of Psychotherapy*. The Johns Hopkins University Press, London.

Glenister, D. & Tilley, S. (1996) Discourse, social exclusion and empowerment. *Journal of Psychiatric and Mental Health Nursing* **3** (19), 3–5.

Goffman, E. (1961) *Asylums*. Peregrine, London.

Goffman, E. (1971) *The Presentation of Self in Everyday Life*. Pelican, London.

Gournay, K. (1995) Mental health nurses working purposefully with people with serious and enduring mental illness – an international perspective. *International Journal of Nursing Studies* **32** (4), 341–352.

Harré, R. (1993) *Social Being*. Basil Blackwell, Oxford.

Harré, R. & Secord, P.F. (1972) *The Explanation of Social Behaviour*. Basil Blackwell, Oxford.

Lipson, M. & Lipson, A. (1996) Psychotherapy and the ethics of attention, *Hastings Center Report* **26** (1), 17–22.

May, D. & Kelly, M.P. (1982) Chancers, pests and poor wee souls: problems of legitimation in psychiatric nursing. *Sociology of Health and Illness* **4** (3), 279–301.

Medico-Psychological Association (1919) *Handbook for Attendants on the Insane*, 6th edn. Bailliere, Tindall and Cox, London.

Mooney, M. (1994) *Vico in the Tradition of Rhetoric*. Hermagoras Press, Davis, California.

Podvoll, E.M. (1990) *The Seduction of Madness: A Compassionate Approach to Recovery at Home*. Century, London.

Robinson, K. (1985) Knowledge and its relationship to health visiting. In *Health Visiting* (K. Luther & J. Orr eds). Blackwell Science, Oxford.

Rogers, B. (1996) Supervised discharge: implications for practice. *Mental Health Nursing* **16** (2), 7–10.

Scheff, T. (1966) *Being Mentally Ill*. Aldine, Chicago.

Shanley, E. (1988) 'Inherently helpful' people wanted. *Nursing Times* **84** (20), 34–35.

Smith, D.E. (1978) 'K is mentally ill': the anatomy of a factual account. *Sociology* **12**, 23–53.

Stanton, A.H. & Schwartz, M.S. (1954) *The Mental Hospital*. Tavistock, London.

Szasz, T. (1979) *The Myth of Psychotherapy: Mental Healing as Religion, Rhetoric and Repression*. Oxford University Press, Oxford.

Tilley, S. (1995a) *Negotiating Realities*. Avebury, Aldershot.

Tilley, S. (1995b) Accounts, accounting and accountability in psychiatric nursing. In *Accountability in Nursing Practice* (Watson R. ed.). Chapman and Hall, Edinburgh.

Wolpert, L. (1995) Descent into darkness. *Guardian*, 17 August 1995, Second Front, p. 2.

Wooff, K. & Goldberg, D. (1988) Further observations on the practice of community psychiatric nurses and mental health social workers. *British Journal of Psychiatry* **153**, 30–37.

11 Negotiating Difference in Mental Health Nursing in New Zealand

Christine Walsh

Introduction

'In the admission and observation ward the ratio was one nurse to five patients with domestic duties given to ward-maids, kitchen-maids, cooks, leaving the nurses free for professional nursing. Remembering my days in Seacliff Hospital in New Zealand, in the 'back ward' where the nurses were forbidden to talk to me (I was told this later by two nurses, now retired), I was amazed to discover that here at the Maudsley it was the nurses' duty to talk to the patients, to get to know them – how else could a correct diagnosis be made?'

(Frame, 1989, p. 373)

The New Zealand writer Janet Frame reminds us that the experience of inpatient hospital care for many patients is dependent on a wide range of variables, not the least of which is location. Mental health nurses work in many different nursing environments world-wide. While the context of nursing may be different, many of the issues arising for nurses working in these different contexts are similar. For example, we all need strategies to deal with the client who is suicidal. However, the strategies we develop and the ways in which these issues are dealt with locally will be different. Recognising difference and taking it into account when relating to clients is a challenge for all nurses working in mental health. The tragedy of mental illness, and its effects on clients and families, demands that nurses work collaboratively towards negotiated outcomes that recognise the uniqueness and diversity of individuals. This is increasingly difficult to achieve in the midst of health reforms which emphasise cost-effective care, which is often focused on the needs of the majority rather than the needs of the person.

One of the most significant policy decisions to influence mental health services has been the drive to move large numbers of clients from institutional care into the community (deinstitutionalisation). These changes have developed through a philosophy of family/community-based care but have been driven largely by the ever-increasing demands on the health care budget. Nowadays in most city streets the legacy of deinstitutionalisation is plain to see: a man standing alone, slightly bent forward, one hand clutching at his trousers trying to hold them up, the other hand gesticulating freely; dishevelled clothing, unshaven, mouth constantly moving, eyes scanning the pavement, shuffling hesitantly forward, keeping to himself. In the past this man probably fitted the criteria for admission to hospital. These days he is a stark reminder of the effects of health care reforms for the mentally ill and policies that have attempted to deal with the perceived needs of the majority.

In this chapter I intend to argue that mental health nurses need to make a commitment to recognising difference and accepting alternative and competing cultural values in the course of their practice, despite pressure to homogenise care. The question and meaning of 'difference' is still being vigorously debated amongst academics, researchers and others.

Feminist academic Carol Bacchi (1990, p. xvi) suggests that the point of reference when debating sameness and difference is always 'man', but she argues that there are limitations with this approach:

'The problem, I suggest, is not men *per se*, but their values and lifestyle. With "man" as the standard for comparison, a claim to "sameness" means aspiring to "masculine" qualities – independence, autonomy, instrumental rationality – and denying one's culturally defined female identity as dependent, emotional and intuitive.'

This desire to replicate the male lifestyle, she claims, is too limiting for women and leaves women with a male-defined identity. Historically the mentally ill have been defined in relation to a point of reference defined by men. This has resulted in some cruel and harsh treatment of women, in particular lesbians, whom therapists tried to cure:

'Albert Ellis, in a 1956 article, reported that through his work with lesbian patients one third were "distinctly improved" and two thirds were "considerably improved" in their progress toward heterosexuality. Ellis explained that his approach was to insist on unmasking the neurotic motivations behind his patients' same-sex love and to show by his manner and verbalisations that he himself was "favourably prejudiced" toward heterosexuality.'

(Faderman, 1991, p. 135)

Difference is not only about other people being different from us, but also about us being different from other people. Central to human interaction is the idea of locating the 'other' (Weedon, 1987). When we are well we locate the 'other' to help us define our own boundaries. When people are unwell their boundaries are often limitless and they rely on professionals to help them to negotiate and set boundaries. Being labelled and treated as mentally ill in itself makes one different, and persons so labelled and treated may need skilled intervention to help them identify who they are and who others are.

It is just as important for the nurse to be able to locate her/his self in order to relate to the client. We locate ourselves in many ways, usually in relation to gender, age or some other category. For white people this also means acknowledging the dominant culture of whiteness (Frankenberg, 1993). In white-dominated societies, white culture can be disregarded while other cultures are considered 'different' and, as such, are visible and therefore commented upon.

From my position as a Pākehā (white) lesbian woman I cannot claim to represent the views of other Pākehā or other lesbians; nor do I claim to speak for Māori. Trying to write about other cultures poses a number of problems for those living outside the culture that they are writing about. One of the problems I have found in writing about Māori is trying to represent specific Māori terms accurately and appropriately. For example the term 'whānau' can have several meanings. It may refer to the nuclear family (uncles, aunts, nieces and nephews), or to a group of people with similar interests such as gangs. In this chapter whānau (family) is defined as 'extended family', an over-simplification of a complex term. I can, however, speak from my experiences and understandings which have developed through being raised in a white culture influenced by traditional western perspectives. I have been further influenced by my training as a nurse, which was shaped largely by conventional western medical practice.

As New Zealand nurses we need to understand that New Zealand is both a bi-cultural and a multi-cultural society. When discussing the relationship between Pākehā (white people) and Māori the term 'bicultural' is used to acknowledge Māori as tangata whenua, 'the people of the land'. This is an important concept to understand because it helps nurses provide appropriate care to Māori and people from other cultures.

In New Zealand the recognition of cultures other than Māori and Pākehā is addressed by the use of the word 'multi-cultural', which is intended to be inclusive of all other cultural groups. However, this situation is not straightforward. Some people may in one instance define themselves as 'Cook Islander' and at another time be prepared to be incorporated under the label 'Māori'. There are no clear lines of demarcation as the choices that people make are often based on the particular situation in which they find themselves. The challenge for nurses then becomes one of facilitation to allow the person to define their own position.

Psychiatric nurses are trained to expect difference in people, to see it and to respond appropriately. Nurses are expected to make 'informed' decisions about these observations. Part of seeking information from the client is an attempt to 'locate' the culture, beliefs, values and ideals of particular clients. This is where the idea of negotiating culture becomes central. Nurses need to acknowledge possible cultural affiliations whilst working to find out how much they matter to the individuals and their families.

It is imperative that nurses working in mental health have an awareness of their own cultural values and how these might have an impact on their relationships with clients, families and colleagues. So the challenge for nurses in this country, and indeed in any country, is to locate their own culture and the culture of the client.

Narratives in research

The stories of experienced psychiatric nurses provide rich and enlightened insights into the complex nature of psychiatric nursing. Of particular value are the descriptions of interactions that demonstrate the use of skills and knowledge in relation to dealing with difference. In addition, nursing stories demonstrate the importance of having an awareness of the environment (including those in the environment and location of the environment) and the appropriate interpretation of multiple cues in order to make informed decisions about nursing care. Two recent New Zealand studies used narratives as part of the research data to illustrate the processes involved in negotiating difference in New Zealand.

The first study, funded by the Health Research Council of New Zealand, examined a new nursing role created with the introduction of the Mental Health (Compulsory Assessment and Treatment) Act on 1 November 1992. During this research, interviews were conducted with 52 experienced mental health nurses from five different centres in New Zealand.

A significant change incorporated in the MH(CAT) Act was the appointment of health professionals to act as duly authorised officers (DAOs). This position is generally held by mental health nurses, although other health professionals have been employed as DAOs. For the first time, aspects of the role of these mental health nurses were legally constituted. DAOs became responsible for co-ordinating the assessment and safeguarding the legal rights of the proposed patient by ensuring that the correct informing processes were followed through, and that accurate documentation was provided (Street & Walsh, 1993).

Of particular interest in this study were findings on the major challenges that nurses, acting in their role as DAOs, faced in dealing with the needs of Māori. Sections 5 and 6 of the Act specifically deal with cultural safety, and many of the nurses interviewed expressed concern at the difficulties of providing a culturally safe service. As researchers we were pleased to have the input of a cultural adviser for this project. Charlene Williams is a Māori of Ngati Toa Rangatira, Raukawa, Tuwharetoa and Rangitane descent and a registered nurse with 30 years nursing experience. It was important to check with Charlene that we were being culturally appropriate throughout the entire project and that our interpretations were sensitive to Māori.

The second study was informed by feminist thought and sought to identify and articulate key issues that nurses saw arising out of their practice as female mental health professionals. In total eight nurses from one centre were interviewed individually, and two focus groups were conducted, to explore the issues and implications for these nurses.

For the purpose of this chapter I have used material from the DAO study to illustrate 'difference' in a cultural context. Material from the second study has been developed to explore gender and 'difference'. Finally I have drawn on personal reflections to raise issues of concern for lesbians in the mental health service.

Cultural contexts

According to a general definition, 'culture is not only a concept which describes the language and way of life of a particular group, but it is also a concept which describes particular groups in relation to others' (Street, 1992a, p. 1). Extending this, it is perhaps useful to recognise that individuals bring their own set of competing cultures into situations. Nurses then respond to cues from the client that help them structure the cultural context in which the nurse and the client interact. When people are unwell the onus of responsibility for detecting the cultural cues remains with the nurse. Therefore nurses should not only have strategies to manage clients with similar cultural beliefs, but also develop ways of working positively and effectively with those whose own cultural beliefs do not match their own.

Nurse theorist Madeleine Leininger has written extensively about the relationship between nursing and culture. In exploring the difference between cultures she states:

> 'Some cultures are strikingly different from others; while other cultures show only slight differences from another culture. The more obvious the cultural differences between particular cultures, the more clearly one can learn to appreciate and understand the concept of culture.'

> (Leininger, 1978, p. 125)

The intersection of the culture of nursing with the medical profession is one example of different cultures in similar contexts. Nursing has been described as a cultural group that is subordinate to the dominant medical culture (Street, 1992b, p. 78). This relationship has its own unique set of power dynamics that rarely change but are sometimes challenged, in particular by nurses, who are seeking to upset the existing order and create a nursing culture that is not controlled by one dominant set of beliefs.

In New Zealand, the term 'cultural safety' has risen to prominence in recent years, particularly in nursing, but is not easily defined. The term developed from efforts to educate nurses to be safe practitioners when nursing people who identify with different cultures and settings (Chapman, 1993). It refers to the nurse's ability to recognise her or his own culture, take into account the culture of other groups, and work towards providing care that respects the differences and similarities. One of the early New Zealand writers at the forefront of discussions on culture, Irihapeti Ramsden, whilst acknowledging the early work of Leininger in the field of cultural difference, had this to say about cultural safety in relation to nursing:

> 'Cultural safety is about power relationships in nursing service delivery. It is also about power relationships between tutors and students of differing cultures. It is about setting up systems which enable the less powerful to genuinely monitor the attitudes and service of the powerful, to comment with safety and ultimately to create useful and positive change which can only be of benefit to nursing and to the people we serve.'

> (Ramsden, 1993, p. 109)

So, it is important to not only acknowledge cultural differences but also to recognise the power relationships that structure these differences.

Māori mental health

Māori make up only 12–15% of the total population of New Zealand. Amongst Māori there are different understandings and adaptations of their own culture. For example in a recent article exploring the changes in Māori society over the past three generations, Bradley (1995, p. 27) suggested that:

> '... Māori whānau (family) are not all the same and that while they are still all Māori they are also dynamic. These differences need to be taken into account when working with whānau in an empowering way.'

A recent report suggests that Māori experience a poorer outcome after their first admission to a psychiatric institution (Te Puni Kokiri, 1993). They are generally hospitalised longer and are much more likely to have subsequent readmissions and hence long-term mental illness. Given the disproportionately high number of Māori among users of the mental health system, this matter is of grave concern.

Throughout the study exploring the new nursing roles created with the Mental Health (Compulsory Assessment and Treatment) Act, Māori argued that their holistic and family/community focus on health was often undermined by the assumptions of the western psychiatric tradition, which is individualised and symptom-based. Durie (cited in Haines, 1987, p. 2) explains that health 'from a Māori perspective, has always acknowledged the unity of the soul, the mind, the body and the family: the four cornerstones of health'.

The mental health public-funded system was originally established to remove people from society. People had a fear of being contaminated by mental disease, or even denied that it existed. These ideas were alien to Māori people whose whānau members suffering from trauma were always included within the tribal networks of whānau (family), hapū (extended family from common ancestors), and iwi (tribe), and given special status (Baker, 1992).

Misinterpretations and misunderstandings

Māori traditions can often be misinterpreted in western medical culture. Māori ways of thinking, speaking, behaving and being have been shaped by a long history and tradition which does not sit comfortably with Pākehā medical structures. Durie (cited in Te Puni Kokiri, 1993, p. 14) suggests two reasons for the reluctance of Māori to enter into hospitalised care:

> 'Firstly, if illness is thought to be related to mākutu or some infringement of tapu, then going to hospital will hardly seem appropriate. Secondly, there may be a high acceptance of abnormal behaviour amongst Māori, leaving illness undetected and untreated.'

The alienation experienced by Māori in institutional care, when separated from whānau (family), hapū (extended family from common ancestors) and iwi (tribe), compounds an already stressful situation for Māori clients and their whānau. This situation is arguably no different for people of different cultures who live in other countries and experience hospitalisation.

Mental health nurses' experiences of work with Māori

As nurses working in the mental health field we are constantly asked to interpret cultural meanings appropriately for any given situation. Listening to nurses speak of their experiences in entering into different cultural environments can help us shape our own cultural and inter-cultural interactions. Furthermore, while we may have some awareness about culture(s), we make judgements about how appropriate it is deal with culture in the specific context. For example, if a person presents in an acute psychotic state the attending nurse may be aware of the cultural needs of the client but may give first priority to the mental health or medical needs. However, sometimes in an acute situation a partial acknowledgement of culture is sufficient to establish rapport. This may be the case regardless of the culture that the nurse identifies with.

In the following account of an acute situation a Māori mental health worker makes the decision that it is not appropriate to start asking the client about his Māori affiliations:

> 'This person was extremely psychotic, he'd been banging his head on the power pole and medically compromised because he did that, and we had to act really different ... and I looked at him and said "kia ora bro" and it was just incredible, it was really difficult to explain, but he could just relate to us, and was just so different.'

The use of language that is specifically Māori ('kia ora' is a greeting in Māori) helped create a way in for this Māori mental health worker to establish some cultural rapport with the client. While the Māori mental health worker has acknowledged and introduced the familiar Māori greeting she has not attempted to go to any exhaustive lengths to assess the specific cultural needs of this client. She has deemed it more important to establish rapport that is aimed at dealing with the client's immediate medical needs.

It is sometimes useful to trace some of the decisions we make about the extent to which we are prepared to incorporate and consider the complex context of culture in our nursing practice. It is often our ability to adapt to competing cultural perspectives that enhances the opportunity to work effectively as nurses.

A Pākehā male nurse, who had trained in Great Britain, describes his encounter with New Zealand culture through his work in a community mental health team:

> 'There was an incident where one of the local elders of the [local Māori] tribe became unwell with no previous history – very well-respected locally, and we were called in. He didn't believe he was unwell and it became really difficult because there were lots of spiritual things going on – being able to look into the future and heal people and that was quite a big issue for me.'

This nurse is faced with having to negotiate competing cultural perspectives. He is influenced by his own 'Anglo Saxon' cultural beliefs and culture, the complex cultural dynamics of nursing and psychiatry, and the cultural perspectives of Māori. In order to work within all these cultural frameworks the nurse has to acknowledge his own limitations and seek the support and expertise of his co-workers. He recognised his anxiety and responded appropriately:

'I was struggling. It was quite frightening, fortunately a Māori mental health worker was available. Again, that makes it difficult because the nature of Māoridom is that everybody knows everybody and has some familial connection. The doctor didn't get around. The situation worked out okay, but it was very hard to do an assessment and maintain cultural safety. I don't know how we get around it.'

By contacting and liaising with the Māori mental health worker, and seeking the guidance and support of that worker, the nurse was able to facilitate a culturally safe environment for that client. This nurse recognised 'difference' in terms of his own culture and that of the client and took the appropriate steps to safeguard both himself and his client. Furthermore he acknowledged the difficulties that dealing with cultural 'difference' poses and the ongoing challenge that this 'difference' generates for nurses who are involved in undertaking nursing assessments in the community.

In small communities, and in particular amongst Māori, there are strong links between families. These links, conveyed by the concept of whānau (family), mean that often the person being assessed or treated is supported and monitored by the whānau. This raises the question of confidentiality of information and client rights. In western medicine ethical frameworks help to structure and control information about clients so that their privacy is protected as much as possible. However, the Māori way of working supports the involvement of whānau in decision making, and lines of communication are clearly not necessarily aligned to next-of-kin status as known in the western world. Involvement of the whānau (family) is problematic if the client does not want the whānau to know their situation or has no desire to have support from the whānau (family).

Alternatively, if the nurse going in to do an assessment is Māori and not related to the family through tribal connections, then the situation calls for a new set of strategies for negotiating entry. Right of entry is not automatic, and the nurse may not be welcomed with open arms. A Māori participant in the study related his experience of moving from one geographical area to another, and spoke of the importance of making the effort to connect with his own tribal affiliations in order to gain acceptance in that particular geographical area:

'What a lot of people don't realise, is that ... it's not just your affiliation when you come to a place, it's what historical affiliations occurred previously to you (in previous generations).'

Fortunately for this nurse the affiliations that he claimed dated back to his great-great-grandfather who is buried close to the side of a local mountain. The relationship that Māori have with the land, and with specific areas of land, is paramount because it provides an affiliation. His ancestral connections sponsored his acceptance into this community through traditional understandings and ceremonies. The time taken by this nurse to acknowledge his tribal affiliations and connections had been well worth the effort:

> 'It's quite funny, I'm actually feeling comfortable here this year. Like last year I wasn't. Each time I'd go out I had to introduce myself quite humbly, but now a lot of the guys are ringing up and saying "We want you to come out here", "na you don't have to be briefed again, you're in" sort of stuff, "your ticket's been punched".'

White nurses working and living in areas with a high Māori population sometimes felt that it was easier for them to negotiate their way into and through encounters with Māori because of the fact that they had experience of either being raised in the local area or living there for quite some time. This, they argued, led to them having more understanding of Māori and being accepted by them so that they could provide a more informed and enlightened cultural perspective to their nursing. However, this view was challenged by other Māori mental health workers, who suggested that it was sometimes very difficult for Pākehā to know when cultural barriers had been breached:

> 'I think people [Pākehā] tend to sort of think "oh well I know these people now" ... but you never know what can blunt people to put them off. You can be very friendly for years and all of a sudden you can insult them on one little point and unless you're aware of it, sometimes that's where they can be really stubborn. Then he's not going to give you anything unless you ask, not even the time of day.'

Thus the possible problems for those nurses working close to cultural groups depended on how and in what ways the particular individual identified with and positioned her or himself in relation to the group. For example a Māori nurse could bring to the encounter both the Māori traditional way of working and the western influences that have been learnt through nursing. Similarly, Pākehā nurses might be influenced by a Pākehā perspective developed through their own socialisation and a Māori perspective influenced through association with Māori.

Negotiating gender in mental health nursing in New Zealand

The issue of how to deal with 'difference' has been, and remains, a challenge to psychiatry. In the second study nurses discussed how gender had an impact on their practice, with most acknowledging that the consideration of gender was an important issue for them, particularly in relation to the diagnosis and treatment of clients. The different ways in which female and male clients were treated raised some interesting questions. How did clinicians take account of gender differences? If they did not, why not? If they did, in what ways was this expressed and what impact did it have on nursing practice and client care?

When gender makes no difference

'Feminism has moved recurrently between the emphasis on equality and the focus on difference; between a politics that points out the irrelevance of sex and insists we should be treated the same, and an alternative that takes sexual difference as its starting point'

(Phillips, 1993, p. 44).

To treat everyone the same, and in this particular case not to consider the impact of gender on nursing practice, is to assume, somewhat naively, that clients want to be responded to and treated in the same way as each other.

One nurse was quite matter-of-fact about her job and did not consider that gender was an issue in her nursing:

'... all I know is that if I'm asked to do a job, to me it doesn't matter if it's a male or a female, I do it. And I don't even think of those sorts of things.'

People's needs often change from moment to moment and this somewhat limited approach falls well short of taking into account any form of difference and therefore the needs of individual clients.

Many of us, regardless of the type of service we are seeking, want our particular needs taken into account, based on our unique circumstances. We expect that the service provider will assess our needs through discussion and communication with us. Recognising the many and varied reasons that bring people to hospital sometimes means looking at different nursing strategies to suit these differences. One nurse described the difficulties of nursing female clients who have been sexually abused:

'I think that it's absolutely imperative that women, if it's appropriate, be nursed by another, if there are psychological, personal or sexuality issues that make it appropriate to be nursed by another woman, then it's appropriate that it should happen.'

This issue seems particularly relevant if the woman client has been sexually abused by a male. The trend these days is to integrate wards so that female and male clients are nursed together. This drive towards 'normalisation' offers less opportunity for 'same gender nursing' though this is sometimes desirable for male as well as female clients.

Differences in diagnosis

A report from the UK (Reaney, 1991), on the ways that women with diagnosed 'personality disorders' have been treated and locked up unnecessarily in 'special hospitals', illustrates the association between diagnosis, treatment and gender.

'Studies have shown that some 48 per cent of women in Britain's three "special hospitals" are categorised as suffering from "psychopathic disorder" as opposed to only 24% of men. "Women are more likely to be sent to a special hospital than men", said Ghandra Gosh, a consultant psychiatrist at maximum security Broadmoor Hospital. "When they transgress social norms they are seen to be more abnormal than a man."'

In the case of personality disorders, the stereotypes typical in our society – that women are passive and sick while men are active and aggressive – contribute to women being diagnosed with dependent personality disorder while men may be diagnosed with antisocial personality disorder (Golden, 1992).

Some nurses in the second study made reference to the ways in which medical staff assigned the label of 'personality disorder' to females and treated them accordingly. One nurse who had started to reflect and research her own practice made the following observations about the treatment of female and male clients:

'A lot of their [female clients'] behaviour in the past, and probably even now, has been seen as "behavioural", "manipulating". But when I sat down and looked at all the males on my caseload, some of them had the same personalities, doing the same type of thing, but that wasn't called behavioural or manipulating. There was a difference in the way that people, you know males in particular, perceived them.'

Recognising the difference in assessment and treatment of her own clients this particular nurse set about devising her own strategies to negotiate this difference:

'And that's something that I'm working quite hard at rectifying. And I'm saying to doctors "why?" I'm questioning it. "Why is she being treated as a personality problem when this guy is doing similar things and he's not a personality problem?" I'm not sure how far I've got with it yet. I guess it's just an awareness thing that I'm coming to.'

This nurse, critiquing and reflecting on her own practice, is now better equipped to discuss difference in the assessment and treatment of her clients when negotiating with medical staff. The next step for this nurse may be to explore the literature surrounding gender so that her negotiations are based on both reflective practice and theoretical perspectives.

Speaking the unspoken: lesbians 'out there'

Another group of women who have been regarded and treated as different based on a particular view of difference are lesbians. Lesbians face difficulties similar to those facing heterosexual women in relation to mental health problems, including depression, anxiety, relationship difficulties, substance abuse, and more serious disorders such as schizophrenia (Perkins, 1995, p. 21).

My experience of working in mental health for 20 years leads me to think that lesbians are minimised and marginalised both as nurses and clients. There have been a number of occasions when I, as a lesbian nurse, have felt sure that a woman client was a lesbian (and I'm certain the client has thought likewise). Unfortunately neither I nor the client has mentioned this to the other because of the unsafe environment and likely backlash to such a disclosure, for both parties. Recently I initiated a conversation with a registered nurse about a client who had self-disclosed as a lesbian. My impression was that this nurse was well aware of the client's sexuality and seemed quite accepting of it. However, in the ensuing conversation with this nurse it was evident that she had very little understanding of the lesbian culture and life style. It is possible that this client would have had to spend a lot of time educating this particular staff member so that her needs could be met, a difficult task for someone mentally unwell. My purpose in pursuing this conversation was to let it be known to staff that I was available for consultation in this matter, just as a Māori or Jewish nurse might make themselves available for a similar reason.

It is difficult to imagine how the mental health service can expect to deal effectively with lesbians when there is little encouragement for lesbians to self-disclose (Hitchcock & Wilson, 1992). In addition to facing many of the 'usual' problems that surround any contact with the mental health service there are many issues that are specific to a lesbian life style that lesbians will not discuss in an unfriendly and 'lesophobic' environment.

When dealing with lesbian clients it is important for the nurse to recognise and acknowledge her or his own relationship with sexual difference. The first step in providing the opportunity for a lesbian to self-disclose is not to assume that all female clients are heterosexual, and instead to respond to any cues that may lead to a lesbian feeling safe to self-disclose. However, it is important to remember that not all lesbians will feel comfortable discussing their sexuality with a male as they may have a mistrust of men based upon previous traumatic experiences. This does not mean that they are man-haters, and the attitude from staff that 'all they need is a good man' does little to enhance a therapeutic relationship, the cornerstone of psychiatric nursing. Some lesbians may not want to self-disclose at all and those that do may ask for this to be kept confidential. All these 'differences' in relation to self-disclosure are part and parcel of recognising that the lesbian culture is as diverse as any other culture.

If nursing staff are to understand some of the issues and therefore 'differences' for lesbians in psychiatric care, they need to recognise that assumptions and 'givens' in mainstream society are not necessarily applicable to lesbian life styles. For example, when asked whom they would like to be notified as the next-of-kin, many lesbians will nominate a partner or close friend and not a blood relative. The blood relative may not be the closest or most appropriate person to be called on and may in fact cause more problems for the client.

Nurses also need to be aware of possible harassment of lesbian clients by male clients and take action to protect lesbians from this. Part of the nurse's response to this could involve setting limits on behaviour from males who do intimidate and harass lesbian clients, while at the same time educating these males about tolerance and acceptance of 'difference'. Recognising that harassment comes from many sources, it is important for nurses to be aware of the actions and behaviour of staff towards lesbian clients. There should be open discussion amongst staff about issues arising for staff in nursing lesbian clients, and educational opportunities for staff to develop strategies to support lesbian clients from an informed and well-balanced perspective.

Conclusion

One of the central themes of this chapter has been the issue of difference and how nurses have assessed and managed difference appropriately. While difference relates to culture, age, ethnicity, sexuality, class and race, in this chapter the focus has been on difference in culture, gender and sexuality.

So what, you might ask, has dealing with difference in New Zealand got to do with mental health nursing in Europe, North America or Asia? How can the nurse working in the mental health area begin to reconcile the complex relationship(s) between the bigger questions of race, sexuality or gender and 'difference' in the face of the ever-changing demands of mental health nursing? All nurses, wherever they are working, should be able to understand, appreciate and care appropriately for clients from different cultural backgrounds. The well-being of the client depends on the extent to which the nurse can understand, accept and manage this.

Nurses should be given the opportunity to extend their knowledge and skills relating to cultural, gender and sexuality differences when working with clients. The nursing curriculum offers such an opportunity for this extension of knowledge. Exploration of themes that target the complex nature of difference should be included in nursing training and in-service training for registered nurses. When negotiating 'difference' in mental health nursing, it may be useful for nurses to consider the client, instead of 'man', as the central reference point. To remain open to such an approach is a challenge not only for nurses, but for any professional working in health care.

Glossary

Aotearoa	New Zealand
hapū	extended family from common ancestor
iwi	tribe; nation; strength
kia ora	good health
mākutu	bewitch; magic; spell
Māori	native New Zealander; belonging to New Zealand
Pākehā	Māori name for white anglocentric people
tapu	forbidden; inaccessible; sacred; not to be defiled
whānau	extended family; be born; family (in a broad sense); offspring

References

Bacchi, C. (1990) *Same Difference: Feminism and Sexual Difference*. Allen & Unwin, Sydney.

Baker, R. (1988) 'Kia Ora Koutou'. In *Psych Nurse's 88* (C. Walsh & S. Johnson eds), Te Ao Maramatanga Conference, Wellington, pp. 37–47.

Bradley, J. (1995) Before you tango with our whānau you better know what makes us tick: an indigenous approach to social work. *Te Komako, Social Work Review* **11** (1), 27–29.

Chapman, A. (1993) The cultural question. *Nursing New Zealand* **1** (5), 31.

Faderman, L. (1991) *Odd Girls and Twilight Lovers: A History of Lesbian Life in Twentieth Century America*. Columbia University Press, New York.

Frame, J. (1989) *Janet Frame: An Autobiography*. Random House, Auckland.

Frankenberg, R. (1993) *White Women, Race Matters: The Social Construction of Whiteness*. University of Minnesota Press, Minneapolis.

Golden, S. (1992) *The Women Outside: Meanings and Myths of Homelessness*. University of California Press, Berkeley.

Haines, H. (1987) *Mental Health For Women*. Reed Methuen, Auckland.

Hitchcock, J. & Wilson, H. (1992) Personal risking: lesbian self-disclosure of sexual orientation to professional health care providers. *Nursing Research* **41** (3), 178–183.

Leininger, M. (1978) *Transcultural Nursing: Concepts, Theories and Practices*. Wily Medical, New York.

Perkins, R. (1995) Meeting the needs of lesbian service users. *Mental Health Nursing* **35** (6), 18–21.

Phillips, A (1993) *Democracy and Difference*. Pennsylvania State University Press, University Park, Pennsylvania.

Ramsden, I. (1993) Kawa whakaruruhau: cultural safety in nursing education in Autearoa (New Zealand). Paper presented to the Second Transcultural Nursing Conference, Cumberland College of Health Sciences, Sydney.

Reaney, P. (1991) Law locks up sane women in Britain. In *The Dominion* (24 March 1991), Wellington.

Street, A. (1992a) *Cultural Practices in Nursing*. Deakin University, Victoria.

Street, A. (1992b) *Inside Nursing: A Critical Ethnography of Clinical Nursing Practice*. State University of New York Press, New York.

Street, A. & Walsh, C. (1993) *Not a Rubber Stamp: Mental Health Nurses Acting as Duly Authorised Officers in New Zealand*. Department of Nursing and Midwifery, Victoria University of Wellington, Wellington.

Te Puni Kokiri (1993) *Nga Ia O Te Oranga Hinengaro Māori. Trends in Māori Mental Health: A Discussion Document*. Ministry of Māori Development, Wellington.

Weedon, C. (1987) *Feminist Practice & Poststructuralist Theory*. Blackwell Science, Oxford.

12 Is Dementia a Challenge to the Identity of the Mental Health Nurse?

Roger Watson

Introduction

I am not trained in psychiatry and not, therefore, strictly speaking a mental health nurse. Nevertheless, I have spent the majority of my time in professional practice caring for people with a mental health problem, namely dementia. For the sake of the present argument, therefore, I will identify myself as a mental health nurse but I realise that this may not accord with everyone's definition. My interest in people with this particular problem has extended into teaching and research and while nobody else has ever questioned my involvement with those suffering from dementia, I have questioned it. In so doing I have also questioned the involvement of others in the care of people with dementia, including the mental health nurse. The question which arises is one of identity and runs along the following lines: cardiac nurses care for people with a cardiac problem, renal nurses care for people with failing kidneys; however, a number of different people care for those suffering from dementia.

Why, therefore, might dementia be a challenge to the identity of the mental health nurse? The simplest answer is that dementia is probably a challenge to the identity, in the professional sense, of anyone who works with those who suffer from this condition. There are several reasons why this might be: dementia care takes place in a number of settings; the very existence of dementia as distinct from the ageing process has been questioned (Berg, 1985); and interventions with people suffering from dementia, while not entirely negligible, are of limited effectiveness.

My experience of people suffering from dementia was gained in a continuing care environment where elderly people with dementing illnesses were cared for alongside others who were cognitively intact. It was not necessary to be trained in mental health nursing to work with elderly people suffering from dementia in this environment and I long held the view that these patients were, somehow, different from those in psychogeriatric and social care. I also assumed that there was a rationale, however tacit, behind the placement of elderly people with dementia in either a continuing care or a psychogeriatric environment.

I now realise that this is not the case and the difficulty for a nurse in understanding the relative placement of elderly people with dementia is further compounded by the placement of elderly people with dementia in social service care. Again, I assumed that a clear rationale would emerge for these placements and, indeed, initial admission to either nursing or social service care is often dictated by the extent of certain physical problems. However, having visited social service homes I was left with the impression that, as nurses, we must disabuse ourselves of the notion that social service care is only for people without significant physical problems. It is not unusual for unqualified staff such as care assistants in social service homes to be dealing with such 'standard' nursing problems as feeding difficulty and incontinence. When I saw others doing what I claimed to be doing, apparently under a different guise, the challenge to my own identity in working with elderly people with dementia began.

Whoever works with elderly people suffering from dementia is involved in living their life for them, to an increasing extent throughout the progression of the disease. The carer becomes not only the eyes, ears and limbs of the person by providing safety, hygiene and nutrition, but also their understanding of the world around them, inasmuch as this is possible, by interpreting cues from the elderly person and also responses to external stimuli such as distress and discomfort. The extent to which any of this is really possible is limited but, nevertheless, it is all being attempted by lay carers, by social service care providers and by mental health and general nurses working with dementia sufferers. A broad spectrum of skills is required and if I have asked myself the question 'What am I doing here?', in relation to my work with dementia sufferers, then I am certain that others, including those trained in mental health nursing, have asked themselves the same question.

The more uncertain I have become about my involvement with dementia sufferers – an uncertainty based on my limited ability to provide for their needs – the more I have studied the conditions which are labelled 'the dementias'. The material which follows is selected from the literature on the history and nature of dementia and the ways in which nurses contribute to the care of dementia sufferers.

As a starting point, and also to illustrate what has been said above, it should be noted that 80% of dementia sufferers are cared for at home. Of the remaining 20%, roughly half are in social service care and half in hospital care, and those in hospital care are roughly equally divided between psychogeriatric and continuing care (Watson, 1993a). Certainly, no group of carers can claim to have a monopoly on caring for people with dementia. In fact, the majority of people with dementia, and some of these are severely demented, are living in the community with their principal carer being a relative or friend. The only group which could be reckoned to have any kind of 'monopoly' of caring for those with dementia is women (Hadfield & Watson, 1994), who are disproportionately represented among those caring for the demented elderly of both sexes in the community.

What is dementia?

The answers to this question are manifold. At the most detached, medico-scientific level, dementia is a progressive global impairment of cognitive function (Council on Scientific Affairs, 1986). This is detached, however, because such a description could never prepare an individual for their suffering of dementia. Nor could it prepare the carer, lay or professional, for the experience of caring for a person who is suffering from dementia. Nevertheless, the description of dementia purely in terms of cognitive decline clearly puts this disorder in the domain of mental health.

However, despite the apparent precision of the description of dementia in terms of cognitive decline, it often obscures the fact that dementia is not a single disorder. Rather, it is the outcome of a number of disease processes, the best known of which is Alzheimer's disease, but the list includes cerebrovascular disease, Pick's disease, Lewy body dementia, Creutzfeldt-Jakob disease and others (Read, 1991). All of these dementing illnesses share incurability and, with the possible exception of cerebrovascular dementia, their origins are obscure.

There is some dispute about the prevalence of Lewy body dementia (Mackay, 1991) and Alzheimer's disease is probably the most common type. However, the distinction between Alzheimer's disease and Lewy body dementia is unclear. The next most common is probably cerebrovascular disease and the other types of dementia. Such epidemiological uncertainties are bound to compromise the identity of nurses working with dementia sufferers because so much of our training depends on a precise diagnosis, albeit that our interest is in the individual's response to their mental health status (the 'subjective experience' referred to by Barker *et al.*, 1995). It is very rarely the case, even with improvements in pre-mortem diagnostic techniques in recent years, that the cause of dementia in an individual is clearly established, with the exception of cerebrovascular occlusion.

Alzheimer's disease and Lewy body dementia are hard to diagnose without a post-mortem examination and the differentiation between types of dementia is a considerable clinical and diagnostic problem (Kukull & Larson, 1989). Alzheimer's disease is the most intensively researched type of dementia and a more detailed look at this condition should help to clarify some of the problems which have arisen in the study of this disease and establish why there are conflicts in and challenges to the identity of the mental health nurse.

The history of dementia

The history of dementia is, essentially, the history of Alzheimer's disease. Though the first description of a disorder which resembled Alzheimer's disease can be dated to 1906 (Berrios, 1990), this does not really date the discovery of the disease which is currently called Alzheimer's disease. Such uncertainty in diagnosing the condition currently labelled

Alzheimer's disease, coupled with the uncertainties referred to above, surely leads all of us involved in the care of those with dementia to ask questions. These questions concern the nature of the condition, the certainty of its diagnosis and the reasons why we are involved at all, and they become even more poignant in attempting to follow the history of dementia to the present day.

The condition which Alois Alzheimer, a German psychiatrist, described in 1906 bore some resemblance to the presently labelled Alzheimer's disease (Berrios, 1990); the person he studied was cognitively impaired and, at post-mortem, the characteristic plaques and tangles which are now taken to be the 'hallmark' of Alzheimer's disease were identified. However, the person, a woman, was young and Alzheimer did not presume to label a new disease. He merely made some observations. The labelling of a condition as Alzheimer's disease came later when Emil Kraepelin, one of Alzheimer's mentors, gave the label to a brain disorder (Berrios, 1990). Nevertheless, it is not clear what the brain disorder thus labelled by Kraepelin was (Watson, 1992a).

Some explanation is required, therefore, for why Alzheimer's disease is now described as the 'silent epidemic' and a major public health problem in the United States and other countries (de Figueiredo, 1993). Quite apart from the obscure origins of Alzheimer's disease and dementia it also has to be taken into account that the condition essentially disappeared for the major part of the century, only to reappear recently described as a major killer. The 'rehabilitation' of Alzheimer's disease from obscurity took about 12 years (Fox, 1989).

Part of the problem was the argument about the distinction between Alzheimer's disease and both previously described dementia and the ageing process itself. Whether or not the ageing process is inevitably associated with memory loss is still in dispute (O'Brien & Levy, 1992). It has to be taken into account that, as the debate has continued, the diagnostic criteria have been sharpened and valid cognitive tests (Folstein *et al.*, 1975; Pfeiffer, 1975) have been developed. Those who diagnose may, as a result, have been enabled to diagnose more of the condition. Alternatively, as Alzheimer's disease is clearly associated with ageing, we may be suffering the consequences of our own success at prolonging life and increasing the number of people attaining greater years. These are perpetual problems for the epidemiologist and the focus of the argument here, while accepting that all of the above may have been operating, will be with the nature of the condition known as Alzheimer's disease. For many years dementia in later life was thought to be inevitable (Fox, 1989). Some people obviously suffered dementia earlier than others but many working in psychiatry and care of the elderly did not recognise the existence of a specific disease leading to catastrophic cognitive decline.

Brain atrophy associated with cognitive decline in relatively young people was recognised as presenile dementia before the recognition of Alzheimer's disease (Anonymous, 1995). The distinction, historically, between Alzheimer's disease and presenile dementia is also unclear. Presenile dementia has been viewed as an early onset of cognitive decline with ageing whereas, and Alzheimer was of this view, Alzheimer's disease was a separate disease (Berrios, 1990).

The situation is no clearer today because the argument now exists between those who view Alzheimer's disease as a separate entity and those (e.g. Brayne & Calloway, 1988) who do not. The latter camp see Alzheimer's disease as an abnormal acceleration of the normal ageing process and there is evidence to support both cases (Von Dras & Blumenthal, 1992).

The plaques and tangles (microscopic neuropathological abnormalities) which are thought to be characteristic of Alzheimer's disease may not be sufficiently characteristic, according to those who see Alzheimer's disease as an acceleration of the normal ageing process. For instance, evidence can certainly be found for the existence of plaques and tangles in the brains of elderly people who have shown no signs of Alzheimer's disease (Fox, 1989). It is now accepted that plaques and tangles may be features of normally ageing brains but the situation regarding their specificity to the characterisation of Alzheimer's disease has now been brought into question.

Relevance to nursing

There are two consequences of the long-standing obscurity of Alzheimer's disease, both having consequences for the mental health nurse. The first of these is that, for the greater part of this century to date, there has been a paucity of research into Alzheimer's disease (Fox, 1989). The argument runs that if a disease does not exist than how can research be conducted into it? The second consequence is: if Alzheimer's disease does not exist, then what is being observed in elderly people with severe cognitive decline? If this is simply ageing, albeit accelerated, then what is the nature of our involvement with it as relatives, psychiatrists, social workers and nurses?

The arguments about research into Alzheimer's disease are possibly relevant to few nurses. This aspect is of more importance to medical researchers, who are ostensibly seeking to understand the condition with a view to a 'cure' for Alzheimer's disease (Deary & Whalley, 1988; Curran, 1989; Grimley Evans, 1992; Doll, 1993; Cordell, 1994). However, knowledge about Alzheimer's disease and knowledge of the debates surrounding this condition are important for nursing. Knowledge helps to form attitudes and attitudes may dictate the way in which we care for people with Alzheimer's disease. It is of passing interest to note that, if Alzheimer's disease is merely an acceleration of the ageing process in the brain, then to effect a cure would be the same as preventing or slowing down the ageing process in the brain (Watson, 1992a). This aspect is also important to those involved in social research because the increasing prevalence of Alzheimer's disease brings with it increasing social problems for the sufferers and for their lay carers (Wattis, 1988; Nygaard, 1991; Baumgarten *et al.*, 1994; Askham, 1995) and also has implications for social policy related to the provision of care (Gray & Fenn 1993; Schneider *et al.*, 1993).

However, the arguments about whether or not Alzheimer's disease is really a distinct disease process or merely an acceleration of an otherwise 'normal' process, e.g. ageing, cannot be ignored by mental health nurses. The reason for this is that our opinion about the nature of Alzheimer's disease will shape our attitude towards those who are suffering from this condition. If we do acknowledge that Alzheimer's disease is really a disease then we are probably more comfortable with the concept of hospitalisation of sufferers and the application of a 'disease' label to them, and we possibly feel more comfortable in the custodial, caring, institutional role which many of us play under these circumstances. Many would see this as leading to negative attitudes towards those with dementia.

If, on the other hand, we view Alzheimer's disease as an accelerated ageing process we may not feel comfortable with the above role. Nevertheless, if we are in the latter camp, there is a still a dilemma and it hinges on whether or not we see senility as an inevitable outcome of ageing or as something which could be prevented. Are those with Alzheimer's disease, in Rowe and Kahn's (1987) terms, 'usual' agers and those without it 'successful' agers? Furthermore, and Goodwin (1991) has been the main proponent of this view, we may fall into the 'myth of senility' trap, whereby we refuse to acknowledge that ageing can lead to significant decline in physical and mental function. As a result, we may begin to judge those who are senile as 'failures'. Viewing someone as a failure may lead to judgemental attitudes and to the wrong therapeutic strategies. According to Goodwin (1991) and Forbes and Hirdes (1993) this is also helping to set a false research agenda into ageing. Few of us acknowledge judgemental attitudes but few of us can deny vain attempts at forcing independence upon elderly people with dementia clearly unable to undertake self-care. Eventually we acknowledge after much personal frustration and induced anxiety in the patient, that such strategies are fruitless.

Goodwin (1991) argues in favour of the 'myth of the myth of senility'. In other words, health care professionals including physicians and nurses, are indoctrinated into believing that senility is a myth. Some believe that, with sufficient prevention, on the one hand, or therapeutic intervention on the other, the adverse effects of ageing can be prevented or alleviated. This may seem like an extreme presentation of one strand of thinking in care of the elderly; nevertheless, it is the guiding philosophy of one school of thought. There is little to guide workers in this area because differentiating between normal and abnormal ageing, between biology and pathology in later life, is still the subject of intense research.

Mental health nurses should therefore recognise, in working with elderly people who are suffering from dementia, that the condition has an obscure history and that, even today, the precise nature of the condition is not fully understood. It is difficult to point to a long tradition in nursing of caring for people with dementia. Even in recent years it is difficult to point to a strand of nursing for people with dementia which is uniquely different from the care delivered by other branches of nursing and social services. Furthermore, if the condition is merely an accelerated or exaggerated form of ageing, then what precisely is the involvement of the mental health nurse? Indeed, it could be argued, what is the involvement of any branch of nursing at all. This latter point is not so hard to address due to the concomitancy of many physical problems such as urinary incontinence (Skelly & Flint, 1995) and inability to carry out activities of daily living, including washing and dressing (Wykle, 1994). These problems do not require the specific skills of the mental health nurse, who is more used to dealing with recognised and often treatable, if not entirely curable, forms of mental illness.

Nursing care of elderly people with Alzheimer's disease

Attention will now be focused on the work of the nurse and others who care for those suffering from dementia. Dementia is characterised by cognitive decline but there are numerous sequelae, including communication problems (Armstrong-Esther & Browne, 1986; Ekman *et al.*, 1991; Burgener & Shimer, 1993), behavioural problems (Teri *et al.*, 1988; Kurita *et al.*, 1993; Näsman *et al.*, 1993), incontinence (Skelly & Flint, 1995), inability to care for oneself (Wykle, 1994), feeding difficulty (Watson, 1993b) and wandering (Hope *et al.*, 1994). The extent to which people suffering from dementia are either disabled or display disordered behaviour in dementia is thought to be largely determined by their cognitive status (Zanetti *et al.*, 1993); and the precise profile of the individual in terms of these problems will depend on the stage of the disease (Cummings & Benson, 1985). For example wandering is characteristic of middle stage Alzheimer's disease and immobility characteristic of late stage; overeating is often observed in the middle stage (Fairburn & Hope, 1988) but in the end stage refusal and/or inability to eat is characteristic (Watson, 1993b). Communication problems make it very difficult, especially in the latter stages, to assess discomfort in elderly people with dementia (Hurley *et al.*, 1992).

The cognitive decline which underlies dementia is arguably why people with this condition come under the care of the mental health services and, specifically, into contact with mental health nurses. One aspect of this decline, behavioural problems, probably falls more in the domain of mental health nurses than any other kind of nursing. These problems can include aggression and sometimes violence (Swearer *et al.*, 1988; Ryden *et al.*, 1991; Patel & Hope, 1992; Aronson *et al.*, 1993; Bridges-Parlet *et al.*, 1994; Malone *et al.*, 1993), antisocial behaviour including sexual problems, such as inappropriate advances and being very demanding towards partners (Haddad & Benbow, 1993a, 1993b), pica (Fisher *et al.*, 1993) and wandering (Hope & Fairburn, 1990). However, what does the mental health nurse have to offer the elderly sufferer with Alzheimer's disease who has behavioural problems?

Interventions with individuals not suffering from Alzheimer's disease but having behavioural problems, are usually aimed at alleviating the problem and even at altering the behaviour of the person on a long-term basis. This is painstaking, highly skilled work which sometimes involves specialist practitioners with qualifications in behavioural therapy. The problem for such approaches when it comes to dementia, is that there is very little evidence that behavioural therapies are of any value. Certainly, aggression and wandering can be managed by chemical restraint in a psychogeriatric environment (Dall, 1995) and in a continuing care environment. If time permits, the wandering person can be accompanied or diverted, but this does not require the specialised skills of a mental health nurse. To all intents and purposes it could be argued that the objective of care in a psychogeriatric environment and in a continuing care environment are identical. Why does one type of care require a mental health nurse and the other not?

Another aspect of cognitive decline is chronic confusion, which is manifested by complete disorientation for time, place and person (Blessed, 1989; Foreman, 1989; Matzo, 1990). The memories of elderly people with dementia become destroyed, their understanding of their environment is reduced or absent and their personality prior to suffering is, essentially, erased. One approach to this aspect of the condition has been the therapeutic approaches involving reminiscence therapy (Woods *et al.*, 1992), reality orientation (Hanley *et al.*, 1981; McMahon, 1988) and validation therapy (Bleathman & Morton, 1988, 1992).

Programmes of physical exercise, and their effectiveness in alleviating problems in dementia (Diesfeldt & Diesfeldt-Groenendijk, 1977) have been studied, as have prospective interventions to alleviate memory deficit (McKitrick *et al.*, 1992). Any carer can carry these out but they are also carried out by specialised therapists. However, the point for the mental health nurse or any other carer/specialist involved in this aspect of care is that there is very little evidence that these strategies work well. Any effects are minimal. This does not mean that they are not worth doing, but do they require the mental health nurse? For example, the best orientation boards and pointers to reality I have observed were in a social service home and not in a hospital.

All of the literature, with regard to the therapeutic interventions referred to above, indicate that there are benefits to be had for individual sufferers and carers alike. Nevertheless – and I have written in favour of continuing research in this area (Watson, 1992b) – it is clear from the literature that any benefits are small. This is particularly true of research on attempts to slow down or reverse cognitive decline, when frequently statistical significance is achieved in comparative or controlled trials, but clinical significance is not yet compatible with wholesale adoption of any therapeutic strategies in the clinical areas.

Finally, in terms of the problems which stem from the cognitive decline in Alzheimer's disease, there are the host of physical problems such as incontinence and feeding difficulty which have been referred to above. These problems certainly do not require the skills and training of a mental health nurse. This is not to classify these problems and nursing responses as basic care (cf. Luikkonen, 1992); rather, they are essential, for example for the maintenance of skin integrity and comfort, although many nurses do not take up the challenge of working with elderly people (Reed, 1989). These problems are not unique to those suffering from dementia, although individuals will suffer from more physical problems if they have dementia.

As dementia progresses all of the above physical problems and problems with activities of daily living become worse. In the terminal stages of the disease, which can last for several years (Norberg *et al.*, 1980), care is almost totally directed at alleviating the effects of these problems, such as pressure sores, skin excoriation and under-nutrition. In a psychogeriatric ward it is very hard to see how the specialist training and skills of the mental health nurse are being used to the full in carrying out this kind of care. It is most unlikely that the mental health nurse entered nursing in order to carry out this 'basic/essential' care and, surely, this must be the time when the identity of the mental health nurse is most greatly challenged. In the terminal stages of dementia the cognitive decline of the Alzheimer's patient is almost complete and there is little therapeutic activity in which the patient, and the mental health nurse, can engage.

Alternative models of dementia care

While passing reference has been made to caring for elderly people with dementia in social services environments, the above account has been mainly concerned with care in environments where nurses, either general or mental health trained, are employed. Future plans for dementia care in the United Kingdom are mainly aimed at bringing this care under the remit of social services and this is particularly exemplified by discussion documents produced in Scotland. These plans are in line both with government plans for care in the community (Griffiths, 1988) and with recommendations by groups such as Scottish Action on Dementia (Killeen, 1991).

Presently, as indicated near the beginning of this chapter, there is little apparent rationale behind the allocation of elderly dementia sufferers to either medical, psychogeriatric or social work care. As the problems of elderly people with dementia who are admitted to social service care worsen, it is possible that they may be transferred to a psychogeriatric or continuing care hospital and may be further transferred between the two. Plans in existence for nearly a decade (Killeen, 1990) have envisaged that dementia care will be planned jointly by social services and health boards in order to maintain people at home for as long as possible. Thereafter, they may be transferred to a home in which social service care and nursing care are both provided under one roof thereby obviating the need to move between institutions. However, in common with plans for community care (Walker, 1995), such plans have been more hoped for than fulfilled and little has changed in the ways of caring for elderly people with dementia.

The concern from the perspective of the mental health nurse is that the type of care currently being delivered is seen as outmoded and inappropriate and there is little specific mention of the nursing component in these, mainly social service oriented, documents. Mental health nurses, already challenged, could be excused for thinking that they are also losing their identity, at least on paper. In countries where such models have been implemented more fully, those who participate in care planning and delivery report on the inappropriateness of nursing care, construed as problem-solving care (Heuke, 1994). Indeed, in these models of care, nurses appear to have been entirely dispensed with.

A more nursing-oriented model of care is being developed and researched in the United States. This is the hospice type of care for elderly people with dementia (Watson, 1994). The main proponent of this type of care is Volicer (Volicer, 1986; Volicer *et al.*, 1986) who has studied extensively the terminal care of elderly people with dementia. His work is now being developed by others (Hanrahan & Luchins, 1995) and it appears that this could be the future direction of dementia care, particularly for those in the terminal stages. There is also considerable discussion in the United States about the requirement for special care units for elderly people with dementia, and hospice type care could be integrated into such units (Berg *et al.*, 1991). Volicer's work is concerned with relief from pain, the indignity of tube feeding in advanced dementia and the parsimonious use of antibiotics in elderly people with dementia. The work looks very promising in terms of valid assessment criteria and models for interdisciplinary teamwork involving relatives and significant others. However, the work is almost entirely aimed at nursing in the general, rather than the mental health, sense. If such a model were to be adopted more widely it would be hard to see how mental health nurses would find a role.

New directions in dementia theory

Most of the literature on dementia paints a very gloomy picture of the prospects for any individual sufferer and for their family. For example, dementia is referred to as 'the never ending funeral' (Fox, 1989); 'a living death' (Wood, 1990); the 'dying of the light' (Anonymous, 1989); 'a disabling neurophysiological disorder' (Richards, 1990); and generally in terms of catastrophe and inevitability. The future for carers who have elderly relatives has been described in terms of 'the worst is yet to come' (Wattis, 1988) and there is much reference in the literature to the concept of 'burden' in relation to dementia (Mangone *et al.*, 1993; Schneider, *et al.*, 1993).

Nevertheless, there is a body of opinion, the main proponent being Kitwood, which proposes a dialectical view of dementia (Kitwood, 1989, 1990, 1993; Kitwood & Bredin, 1992). This view criticises current research and therapeutic strategies and claims that a significant element in the dementia of, for example, an Alzheimer's disease sufferer, is socially constructed. This approach claims that a degree of 'rementia' should logically be possible if the socially constructed factors can be identified, isolated and neutralised through alternative therapeutic strategies. Where does this thinking lead the mental health nurse? Does the current practice of mental health nurses actually encourage or accelerate the dementing process and is the possibility of 'rementia' acknowledged within mental health nursing?

The optimistic paradigm in dementia care

Closely related to the above and, to some extent, interrelated with it, is a new paradigm developing in dementia care. I call this the 'optimistic paradigm' because it directly challenges the burden paradigm which has dominated thinking in dementia care for the past few decades. Burden, as a concept, has been reviewed by Warnes (1993) who says that there is considerable confusion about application of the concept of burden to the sufferer, the carers, or the state. Moreover, it has very negative connotations as those who are considered to be a burden are also considered to be a 'nuisance' and to cost 'excessive' amounts of money (Warnes, 1993). However, recalling my question above on the ideas of rementia, I wonder if this new paradigm has anything to offer nurses who work with elderly people who are suffering from dementia.

What does the optimistic paradigm say? According to its adherents, who were much in evidence at the quadrennial III European Congress of Gerontology in 1995 (LeNavanec, 1995; Swane, 1995; Miesen, 1995), there should be other ways of assessing the impact of dementia on individuals and families; there must be positive as well as negative aspects to dementia and we must recognise the 'personhood' and the individuality of those suffering from dementia. I feel that taking into account the potential for positive aspects of dementia is challenging for health care practitioners, and nurses in particular, because it is the nature of our work as nurses to approach things from a problem-led perspective; within the burden paradigm.

I see an imbalance in these two perspectives. On the one hand those of us who could be accused of being 'burdened by the burden paradigm' are always hoping that there is some glimmer of individuality, of personhood, in those for whom we care and who we involve in our research. It is my estimation that we are willing to acknowledge signs of hope despite our own tendency to see things from a problem-led perspective. On the other hand, there is an element of intolerance within the optimistic paradigm which now tends to dismiss any talk of burden or problem in dementia. It turns its back on research and teaching which, while they may or may not come from within the burden paradigm, certainly come from people who are recognised as working within that paradigm, nurses being a classic example.

This is where the challenge lies: the retort from those of us who have been 'burdened' until now should be 'What is the evidence for accepting a new paradigm?'. The most difficult issue is not acceptance; rather, the problem lies in rejection of the old paradigm of burden, for which the evidence (some presented above) is copious. I am not so naïve as to suppose that these paradigms can rest comfortably side-by-side and, while they may not immediately change the everyday practice of nurses working with elderly people who are suffering from dementia, they may alter the research agenda in the social sciences. The medical and biological research agenda, which seeks an explanation and a cure, will be relatively immune to this. However, research which aims to improve the care of elderly people with dementia through the alleviation of their problems and their carers' burdens may be usurped by the optimistic paradigm. It is too early to say what the alternative research agenda would be and it is clearly impossible to predict where it will lead.

Summary and conclusions

Some of the potential challenges to the identity of nurses working with elderly people who are suffering from dementia have been presented. These include the fact that there are some doubts about the existence of dementia as a disease process distinct from the process of ageing, and this raises the problem for those in mental health of what it is that they are doing.

The progressive and incurable nature of dementia sets it aside from most other mental health illnesses. It is a condition from which there is no remission and no prospect of a return to 'normality' or the previous mental state of the sufferer. This alone, of course, does not preclude dementia care from the nursing realm but, with a specific view to mental health nursing, where therapies are often applied in order to alleviate conditions, there is very little evidence of the effectiveness of any therapeutic approaches to dementia. Again, the role of the mental health nurse is brought into question.

The predominance of physical problems in the terminal stages of dementia is probably a major challenge to the identity of the mental health nurse. Dealing with the heavy physical work involved in attending to the essential needs of heavily dependent individuals is, arguably, not the work of the mental health nurse. Many must feel that their true 'calling' and interpersonal skills are being wasted. The other side of the coin is that nurses in general nursing continuing care environments surely see this aspect of dementia care as their work. Furthermore, the other people, such as care assistants and others in both nursing and social work who are involved in caring for elderly people with dementia, have to be considered.

The above challenges to the identity of the mental health nurse arise on the basis of comparison with other caring professionals. However, as described towards the end of this chapter, more fundamental challenges to the whole notion of nursing care, especially as a problem-oriented practice, are appearing on the horizon. These will challenge the identity, not only of the mental health nurse, but of all nurses involved in the care of elderly people with dementia. This latest, and potentially most serious, challenge to nursing practice in the area of dementia care comes from outside the profession; from psychologists, sociologists and others who have an interest in dementia. It is often the case that these other professions encounter dementia sufferers at an earlier stage of the dementing process than nurses do. Could it be the case that they rarely witness the extreme debilitation of the later stages? Is there a reluctance on their behalf to admit failure and the fact that the point inevitably arises when many dementia sufferers have to be 'handed over' to a more intensive kind of caring environment? If we acquiesce too readily to the new paradigm in dementia care we may be discarding prematurely anything that is of value in the nursing care of people with dementia; we may, in fact, be doing those individuals who suffer, and their families, a great disservice.

There are issues relevant to learner nurses, inasmuch as they need to be properly prepared for the multi-faceted approach to dementia care which they will encounter in practice. Mental health nurses need to be educated so that they appreciate their role in caring for elderly people with dementia alongside other professionals within and outside of nursing. For nurse educators, those parts of the curriculum related to care of elderly people with dementia possibly need to be reconsidered. On the one hand there is a wide range of scientific knowledge to be conveyed about the care of elderly people with dementia and, on the other hand, there is the moral commitment to caring for people who are irreversibly and increasingly cognitively impaired. If the right balance is struck between the scientific and the moral dimensions, then learner nurses will be enabled adequately to appraise the arguments from those who see dementia from different perspectives.

References

Anonymous (1989) The dying of the light. *The Economist* 23 September 1989, 145–146.

Anonymous (1995) Dementia through the ages: an historical overview. *The Karger Gazette* **55**, 5.

Armstrong-Esther, C.A. & Browne, K.D. (1986) The influence of elderly patients' mental impairment on nurse–patient interaction. *Journal of Advanced Nursing* **11**, 379–387.

Aronson, M.K., Cox Post, D. & Guastadisegni, P. (1993) Dementia, agitation, and care in the nursing home. *Journal of the American Geriatrics Society* **41**, 507–512.

Askham, J. (1995) Making sense of dementia: carers' perspectives. *Ageing and Society* **15**, 103–114.

Barker, P.J., Reynolds, W. & Ward, T. (1995) The proper focus of nursing: a critique of the 'caring' ideology. *International Journal of Nursing Studies* **32**, 387–397.

Baumgarten, M., Hanley, J.A., Infante-Rivard, C., Battista, R.N., Becker, R. & Gauthier, S. (1994) Health of family members caring for elderly persons with dementia. *Annals of Internal Medicine* **120**, 126–132.

Berg, L. (1985) Does Alzheimer's disease represent an exaggeration of normal ageing? *Archives of Neurology* **42**, 737–739.

Berg, L., Buckwalter, K.C., Chafetz, P.K. *et al.* (1991) Special care units for persons with dementia. *Journal of the American Geriatrics Society* **39**, 1229–1236.

Berrios, G.E. (1990) Alzheimer's disease: a conceptual history. *International Journal of Geriatric Psychiatry* **5**, 355–365.

Bleathman, C. & Morton, I. (1988) Validation therapy with the demented elderly. *Journal of Advanced Nursing* **13**, 511–514.

Bleathman, C. & Morton, I. (1992) Validation therapy: extracts from 20 groups with dementia sufferers. *Journal of Advanced Nursing* **17**, 658–666.

Blessed, G. (1989) Managing dementia. *Journal of District Nursing* **7** (10), 4–6.

Brayne, C. & Calloway, P. (1988) Normal ageing, impaired cognitive function, and senile dementia of the Alzheimer's type: a continuum? *The Lancet* **331** (8597), 1265–1266.

Bridges-Parlet, S., Knopman, D. & Thomson, T. (1994) A descriptive study of physically aggressive behaviour in dementia by direct observation. *Journal of the American Geriatrics Society* **42**, 192–197.

Burgener, S.C. & Shimer, R. (1993) Variables related to caregiver behaviours with cognitively impaired elders in institutional settings. *Research in Nursing and Health* **16**, 193–202.

Council on Scientific Affairs (1986) Dementia. *Journal of the American Medical Association* **256**, 2234–2238.

Cordell, B. (1994) β-amyloid formation as a potential therapeutic target for Alzheimer's disease. *Annual Review of Pharmacology and Toxicology* **34**, 69–89.

Cummings, J.L. & Benson, D.F. (1985) Which symptoms of dementia point to Alzheimer's? *Diagnosis* **7** (11), 36–50.

Curran, S. (1989) Round up: searching for the cause of Alzheimer's disease. *Geriatric Medicine* **19** (3), 13–14.

Dall, J. (1995) Practical management of elderly patients with intellectual loss. *Karger Gazette* **55**, 6–7.

de Figueiredo, J.M. (1993) Epidemiology of Alzheimer's disease: research trends in the United States. *International Journal of Geriatric Psychiatry* **8**, 59–65.

Deary, I.J., & Whalley, L.J. (1988) Recent research on the causes of Alzheimer's disease. *British Medical Journal* **297**, 807–810.

Diesfeldt, H.F.A. & Diesfeldt-Groenendijk, H. (1977) Improving cognitive performance in psychogeriatric patients: the influence of physical exercise. *Age and Ageing* **6**, 58–64.

Doll, R. (1993) Review: Alzheimer's disease and environmental aluminium. *Age and Ageing* **22**, 138–153.

Ekman, S.L., Norberg, A., Viitanen, M. & Winblad, B. (1991) Care of demented patients with severe communication problems. *Scandinavian Journal of Caring Sciences* **5**, 163–170.

Fairburn, C.G. & Hope, R.A. (1988) Changes in eating in dementia. *Neurobiology of Ageing* **9**, 28–29.

Fisher, J.E., Fink, C.M. & Loomis, C.C. (1993) Frequency and management difficulty of behavioural problems among dementia patients in long-term care facilities. *Clinical Gerontologist* **13**, 3–12.

Folstein, M.F., Folstein, S.E. & McHugh, P.R. (1975) 'Mini-mental state': a practical method for grading the cognitive state of patients for the clinician. *Journal of Psychiatric Research* **12**, 189–198.

Forbes, W.F. & Hirdes, J.P. (1993) The relationship between ageing and disease: geriatric ideology and myths of senility. *Journal of the American Geriatrics Society* **41**, 1267–1271.

Foreman, M.D. (1989) Confusion in the hospitalised elderly: incidence, onset, and associated factors. *Research in Nursing and Health* **12**, 21–29.

Fox, P. (1989) From senility to Alzheimer's disease: the rise of the Alzheimer's disease movement. *Millbank Quarterly* **67**, 58–103.

Gray, A. & Fenn, P. (1993) Alzheimer's disease: the burden of illness in England. *Health Trends* **25**, 31–37.

Goodwin, J.S. (1991) Geriatric ideology: the myth of the myth of senility. *Journal of the American Geriatrics Society* **39**, 627–631.

Griffiths, R. (1988) *Community Care: Agenda for Action*. HMSO, London.

Grimley Evans, J. (1992) From plaque to placements; a model for Alzheimer's disease. *Age and Ageing* **21**, 77–80.

Haddad, P.M. & Benbow, S.M. (1993a) Sexual problems associated with dementia:

Part 1: Problems and their consequences. *International Journal of Geriatric Psychiatry* **8**, 547–551.

Haddad, P.M. & Benbow, S.M. (1993b) Sexual problems associated with dementia: Part 2. Aetiology, assessment and treatment. *International Journal of Geriatric Psychiatry* **8**, 631–637.

Hadfield, N. & Watson, R. (1994) Alzheimer's disease: who cares? *Elderly Care* **6** (2), 14–16.

Hanley, I.G., McGuire, R.J. & Boyd, W.D. (1981) Reality orientation and dementia: a controlled trial of two approaches. *British Journal of Psychiatry* **138**, 10–14.

Hanrahan, P. & Luchins, D.J. (1995) Access to hospice programs in end-stage dementia: a national survey of hospice programmes. *Journal of the American Geriatrics Society* **43**, 56–59.

Heuke, M. (1994) Communication assessment scales. Alzheimer's disease. Xth International Conference, 21–23 September, Edinburgh.

Hope, R.A. & Fairburn, C.G. (1990) The nature of wandering in dementia: a community-based study. *International Journal of Geriatric Psychiatry* **5**, 239–245.

Hope, R.A., Tilling, K.M., Gedling, K., Keene, J.M., Cooper, S.D. & Fairburn, C.G. (1994) The structure of wandering in dementia. *International Journal of Psychiatry* **13** (9), 149–155.

Hurley, A.C., Volicer, B.J., Hanrahan, P.A., Houde, S. & Volicer, L. (1992) Assessment of discomfort in advanced Alzheimer's patients. *Research in Nursing and Health* **15**, 369–377.

Killeen, J. (1990) *Dementia: Sharpening Local Plans. Priorities for the '90s.* Scottish Action on Dementia, Edinburgh.

Killeen, J. (1991) *Dementia in Scotland. Agenda for action.* Scottish Action on Dementia, Edinburgh.

Kitwood, T. (1989) Brain mind and dementia: with particular reference to Alzheimer's disease. *Ageing and Society* **9** 1–15.

Kitwood, T. (1990) The dialectics of dementia: with particular reference to Alzheimer's disease. *Ageing and Society* **10**, 177–186.

Kitwood, T. (1993) Towards a theory of dementia care: the interpersonal process. *Ageing and Society* **13**, 51–67.

Kitwood, T. & Bredin, K. (1992) Towards a theory of dementia care: personhood and well-being. *Ageing and Society* **12**, 269–287.

Kukull, W.A. & Larson, E.B. (1989) Distinguishing Alzheimer's disease from other dementia: questionnaire responses of close relatives and autopsy results. *Journal of the American Geriatrics Society* **37**, 521–527.

Kurita, A., Blass, J.P., Nolan, K.A., Black, R.S. & Thaler, H.T. (1993) Relationship between cognitive status and behavioural symptoms in Alzheimer's disease and mixed dementia. *Journal of the American Geriatrics Society* **41**, 732–736.

LeNavenec, C. (1995) Understanding the social context of families experiencing dementia: a qualitative approach. III European Congress of Gerontology, 30 August to 2 September 1995, Amsterdam.

Luikkonen, A. (1992) Basic care of demented patients living in institutions. *Journal of Clinical Nursing* **1**, 345–350.

Mackay, A. (1991) Subtypes of dementia. Scottish Action on Dementia Annual Conference, Glasgow, 24 June 1991. Scottish Action on Dementia, Edinburgh.

Malone, M.L., Thomson, I. & Goodwin, J.S. (1993) Aggressive behaviours among institutionalised elderly. *Journal of the American Geriatrics Society* **41**, 853–856.

Mangone, C.A., Sanguinetti, R.M., Bauman, P.D. *et al.* (1993) Influence of feelings of burden on the caregiver's perception of the patient's functional status. *Dementia* **4**, 287–293.

Matzo, M. (1990) Confusion in older adults: assessment and differential diagnosis. *Nurse Practitioner* **15** (9), 32–46.

McKitrick, L.A., Camp, C.J. & Black, F.W. (1992) Prospective memory intervention in Alzheimer's disease. *Journal of Gerontology* **47**, 337–343.

McMahon, R. (1988) The '24-hour reality orientation' type of approach to the confused elderly; a minimum standard for care. *Journal of Advanced Nursing* **13**, 693–700.

Miesen, B.M.L. (1995) Awareness in Alzheimer's disease patients: consequences for research and caregiving in dementia. III European Congress of Gerontology, 30 August to 2 September 1995, Amsterdam.

Näsman, B., Bucht, G., Eriksson, S. & Sandman, P.O. (1993) Behavioural symptoms in the institutionalised elderly – relationship to dementia *International Journal of Geriatric Psychiatry* **8**, 843–849.

Norberg, A., Norberg, B. & Bexell, G. (1980) Ethical problems in feeding patients with advanced dementia. *British Medical Journal* **281**, 847–849.

Nygaard, H.A. (1991) Who cares for the caregiver? *Scandinavian Journal of Caring Science* **5**, 157–162.

O'Brien, J.T. & Levy, R. (1992) Age associated memory impairment. *British Medical Journal* **304**, 5–6.

Patel, V. & Hope, R.A. (1992) A rating scale for aggressive behaviour in the elderly – the RAGE. *Psychological Medicine* **22**, 211–221.

Pfeiffer, E. (1975) A short portable mental status questionnaire for the assessment of organic brain deficits in elderly patients. *Journal of the American Geriatrics society* **23**, 433–441.

Read, S. (1991) In *Comprehensive Review of Geriatric Psychiatry* (J. Sadavoy, L.W. Lazarus & L.F. Jarvik eds). American Psychiatric Press, Washington, pp. 287–310.

Reed, J. (1989) All dressed up and nowhere to go. Poster displayed at Royal College of Nursing Research Advisory Group Conference, 14–16 April 1989, Swansea.

Richards, B.S. (1990) Alzheimer's disease: a disabling neurophysiological disorder with complex nursing implications. *Archives of Psychiatric Nursing* **4**, 39–42.

Rowe, J.W. & Kahn, R.L. (1987) Human ageing: usual and successful. *Science* **237**, 143–149.

Ryden, M.B., Bossenmaier, M. & McLachlan, C. (1991) Aggressive behaviour in cognitively impaired nursing home residents. *Research in Nursing and Health* **14**, 87–95.

Schneider, J., Kavanagh, S., Knapp, M., Beecham, J. & Netten, A. (1993) Elderly people with advanced cognitive impairment in England: resource use and costs. *Ageing and Society* **13**, 27–50.

Skelly, J. & Flint, A.J. (1995) Urinary incontinence associated with dementia. *Journal of the American Geriatrics Society* **43**, 286–294.

Swane, C.E. (1995) Dementia and dehumanisation: everyday life experiences. III European Congress of Gerontology, 30 August to 2 September 1995, Amsterdam.

Swearer, J.M., Drachman, D.A., O'Donnel, E.F. & Mitchell, A.L. (1988) Troublesome and disruptive behaviours in dementia: relationships to diagnosis and disease severity. *Journal of the American Geriatrics Society* **36**, 784–790.

Teri, L., Larson, E.B. & Reifler, B.V. (1988) Behavioural disturbance in dementia of the Alzheimer's type. *Journal of the American Geriatrics Society* **36**, 1–6.

Volicer, L. (1986) Need for hospice approach to treatment of patients with advanced progressive dementia. *Journal of the American Geriatrics Society* **34**, 655–658.

Volicer, L., Rheaune, Y., Brown, J., Fabiszewski, K. & Brady, R. (1986) Hospice approach to the treatment of patients with advanced dementia of the Alzheimer type. *Journal of the American Medical Association* **16**, 2210–2213.

Von Dras, D.D. & Blumenthal, H.T. (1992) Dementia of the aged: disease or atypical accelerated ageing? Biopathological and psychological perspectives. *Journal of the American Geriatrics Society* **40**, 285–294.

Walker, A. (1995) *Half a Century of Promises*. Counsel and Care, London.

Warnes, A.M. (1993) Being old, old people and the burdens of burden. *Ageing and Society* **13**, 297–338.

Watson, R. (1992a) Alzheimer's disease: does it exist? *Nursing Standard* **6** (43), 29–31.

Watson, R. (1992b) Is elderly care research-based? *Nursing Standard* **6** (48), 37–39.

Watson, R. (1993a) *Caring for Elderly People*. Baillière Tindall, London.

Watson, R. (1993b) Measuring feeding difficulty in elderly patients with dementia: perspectives and problems. *Journal of Advanced Nursing* **18**, 25–31.

Watson, R. (1994) Towards a more compassionate model of care. *Journal of Dementia Care* **2** (6), 18–19.

Wattis, J.P. (1988) Caring for the demented: the worst is yet to come. *Geriatric Medicine* **18**(5), 69–73.

Wattis, J.P. (1988) Dementia means the carer goes to bed angry. *Geriatric Medicine* **18** (7), 40–41.

Wood, C. (1990) A living death. *Community Outlook* June 30–32.

Woods, B., Portnoy, S. Head, D. & Jones, G. (1992) Reminiscence and life review with persons with dementia: which way forward? In *Care-giving in Dementia* (G. Jones & B.M.L. Miesen eds). Routledge, London, pp. 137–161.

Wykle, M.L. (1994) Nursing care in Alzheimer's disease. *Clinics in Geriatric Medicine* **10**, 351–365.

Zanetti, O., Bianchetti, A., Frisoni, G.B., Rozzini, R. & Trabucchi, M. (1993) Determinants of disability in Alzheimer's disease. *International Journal of Geriatric Psychiatry* **8**, 581–586.

Conclusion

Stephen Tilley

An excursion to Duns

Recently, at mid-afternoon in a Scottish town called Duns, I saw a man stand addressing the town square and anyone who listened. The man in the square – next to him stood a woman who said nothing – repeatedly emphasised his main point: the King James version of the Bible was the only correct version, and to read or follow any other version would be highly pernicious and dangerous (for the soul or spirit).

Several people stood at different distances and listened. A couple of young men walked by mocking the man, but did not linger to hurt or further insult him. A man near me kept turning to me to question or subvert something the man had said. But mainly the people listened.

I wondered how long the man in the square would go on, and how long the others' tolerance of his claiming the space of the square would last. I wondered if they might see him as a crank, or mad. When I left, the man was still speaking, and folk remained.

This episode seemed somehow linked to this book. In particular, it raised questions about texts, about their possible canonical status, about 'the book' or 'the Book', and the relationship of text to practice. Britain, and Scotland, are not innocent with regard to struggles over texts and their truth. In the part of Scotland around Duns, wars have been fought over interpretations of biblical texts and their implications. Differences between people were marked by references to texts and different interpretations of texts.

However, this raises a new set of problems. Though people were all 'people of the Book', their differences among themselves forced the questions: Which book? Which version of *the* Book? If there is not *a* book, or Book, which can be agreed to be the source of truth, then the basis for regarding ourselves as a people, or the people, might be at risk. The quest for an authorised version, the meaning of which is set and available to all at all times, necessitates preserving the authority of the text and assuring interpreters' fidelity to it as the source of truth.

Today British mental health nursing is a contested realm. Small scale 'care wars' are being waged, in texts about what care is, how central it is and who deserves it – the focus, scope and intention of psychiatric nursing. Debates and arguments in mental health nursing journals mark the emergence of defensible positions and claims about appropriate knowledge, incipient 'schools' of mental health nursing. To a greater extent than before, what is true about psychiatric and mental health nursing, and what the rights and obligations of the psychiatric and mental health nurse are in the light of that truth, are contested matters.

Clearly the 'care wars' are not literal counterparts to past controversies and wars over religious doctrine and practice. Nonetheless, there is a parallel issue. In the 'care wars', debate sometimes centres on the search for an authorised version or canonical text. Thus, in a set of recent articles, the relevance of theories and models for mental health nursing practices was disputed, with specific reference to the value of Peplau's work (Reynolds & Cormack, 1990; Gournay, 1995; Barker & Reynolds, 1996), and the value of Peplau's work, compared to a putative 'ideology of caring', was asserted (Barker *et al.*, 1995).

This book is not a salvo in the 'care wars'. The text began with an argument for allowing each nurse to present her or his own 'version' of the mental health nurse. The argument, referring to recent literary theory, may have seemed slightly defensive, almost an excuse for alluding to literary matters when considering issues of practice. But at this point, on the basis of the texts in this book, it is quite appropriate to justify attention to the importance of language in use – in current parlance, 'discourses' – in considering the worlds that mental health nurses and patients inhabit and shape.

In considering those worlds, we must be struck by how different they are. This book is not a chorus, but a set of voices. Each voice tries to make space for a version of the mental health nurse, but does not aim to exclude all others. Nor is there an over-riding editorial/authorial voice, ordering and regulating the other voices. While the reader may detect the potential for the voices to dispute among themselves (for example, over whether the subject is the 'mental health nurse' or the 'psychiatric nurse' or the 'mental nurse'), the texts, individually and collectively, do not try to present a single authoritative version of the nurse. It is not a single canonical text. Instead, each contribution is open for response, and the effect of them all is to construct a space open for more and different versions of the mental health nurse.

Response and responsibility

The above account may downplay the problems of speaking and responding, finding voice and space to articulate one's views. A number of the contributors note some of those problems: gender-structured inequalities of opportunity to speak and respect for views (Gallop); privileging of a psychiatric, or of a particular psychiatric nursing, point of view (Parkes, Ritter); uncertainty about what one is doing (Tilley); repression (Glenister); bearing silence (Altschul); doubt about the legitimacy of one's position, and structures of power permeating talk in practice and in the classroom (Ritter).

But the contributors to this book suggest that it is possible, if not easy, to take part in the processes and struggles outlined above. According to my reading, all of the authors construct, explicitly or implicitly, the mental health nurse as a person who must take personal responsibility for addressing those problems in situations of face-to-face interaction with people with mental illness, for seeking to change the conditions which distort and inhibit communication and interaction, and for being aware of the nurse's part in perpetuating those conditions. Some suggest the relevance of specific kinds of knowledge; in particular, knowledge of the workings of power, as structured institutionally and in interpersonal relations, and sociological thinking on the construction of deviance.

Assuming this responsibility is not straightforward. The mental health nurse is strongly bound by, and reflexively participates in constructing, various contexts – institutional, social, cultural and political contexts – which condition the possibilities presented by the contributors. Among the possibilities are:

(1) that the MHN can confront his or her own capacity for coercion and control of others regarded as mentally ill; can recognise how in doing so he/she takes part in, and reproduces, wider patterns of coercion and control; and thus can gain the possibility of changing these relationships, with their damaging impact on patients and nurses;

(2) that the MHN can become aware of the way difference operates in interpersonal and intergroup relations, distancing the differentiating other, and rendering him/them unknown, or knowable only as 'other', 'not like me';

(3) that the MHN can use her or his own personal experience to relate to people others find difficult, in the coffee-and-cigarette-and-time-together realm of everyday life;

(4) that the MHN can recognise male psychiatrists' limitations in relating to and caring for women patients; and

(5) that the MHN can work to ensure that patients come first.

Thus, to see the mental health nurse as responsible for change is to adopt a radical perspective, and to set a radical agenda (or radical agendas) for mental health nursing practice and education.

Themes from the book

The texts can be read as responses to implicit questions: 'Who am I?/ Who is the mental health nurse?' and 'How have I come to be as I am?/ How does one become a mental health nurse?'. Some general themes related to mental health nursing, and to accounting for oneself as a nurse, can be picked out:

(1) The mental health nurse is a person encountering people with mental illness and being attracted to them – to their 'human peculiarities', or to some perceived conundrum: Why do they keep poisoning themselves? The responses of the nurses, once in relation to the patient, include: research and science as one way to answer questions about the relationship and

interaction; the nurse's moves, in thinking and being, and literally from job to job, in an effort to find a way to relate personally to patients; and involvement in management or in group work. And what qualities do the contributors suggest are needed? Some note the need for 'ego strength', or the ability to manage tensions; ability to tolerate silence; willingness to recognise issues of coercion and control; and capacity to tolerate and use the negative or ambivalent quality of relationships. Thus the personal experience of engagement and involvement with patients may have, for different nurses, a number of different sequelae.

(2) There is tension in the varied knowledge and information appropriate for mental health nursing practice; between nursing science, art, and what Barker and Whitehill (this volume) call 'craft'. The chapters taken together indicate that the authors would neither disregard science, nor caricature it as inhuman, dehumanising or reductionist, but would rather envision the possibilities of a science that is human and humanly motivated. Such a science would be suitable for informing practice shaped by sensitivity to the politics of the psychiatric institutions, and sensitivity to the particular philosophical problems posed by the experience of mental illness (e.g. the problem of the 'neurotic' patient's responsibility). The science, the art and the craft of mental health nursing represented in this volume, are all forms of response by these contributors to their involvement in situations of care with or for people experiencing mental illness in particular settings. The contributors have learned through experience (e.g. Tennant, Parkes and Altschul), through systematic enquiry and literature review (Gallop, Ritter, Walsh, Glenister and Watson), through metaphorical extension (Ryan, and Tilley), through further study in different fields (Pollock), and through dialogue and collaborative investigation (Barker and Whitehill).

(3) There is an ambiguous quality to the contributors' narratives of experience. What comes through most strongly is the strong sense of the nurse as self-as-actor, that is, the reflexive practitioner moving through experience, engaged with other and self. However, in most of these chapters, fundamental ambiguities set up tensions. These tensions can be discerned in the 'ratios' of the elements in contributors' narratives; the elements of actor, means, act, setting and motive (Burke, 1969)*. Which element of the narrative is particularly ambiguous and problematic differs in the various accounts: in some, the act is ambiguous (Tilley), in some it is the motive (Glenister's care or coercion; Ritter's nurses questioning the legitimacy of psychiatrists' authority and power). The relationship between actor and means, between agent and agency may be problematic. Is the patient the means the nurse uses to accomplish some goal set by society or by psychiatry? Is the nurse the means the patient uses to achieve her or his self-defined ends (Barker and Whitehill)? The definition of the actor may be problematic (nurses, like patients, as women – Gallop, Parkes). The setting (practice or educational) may be ambiguous or problematic (the inpatient

---

* See Tilley (1995a, 1995b) for an account of narrative analysis based on these elements of Burke's 'dramatist pentad'.

setting, in Tennant; or, for Walsh, culture; for Ryan, the conjunction of educational and practice settings).

(4) The contributors' narratives belong to different genres. The 'plot' may be 'career' (Parkes, Gallop, Pollock); it may be ironic (Tennant's battle or picaresque adventure, Parkes' vision of the quixotic mental health nurses banished from their castles); or it may depend on a metaphorical shift (Tilley's nurse as rhetorician; Ryan's amphibian nurse, teacher or researcher) or metonymic extension (Walsh's differences of culture, gender, or sexual orientation, and New Zealand differences generally, stand for a wider 'difference'); it may involve a philosophical deepening (Ryan's layering of ambiguities; Ritter's, or Watson's, or Glenister's uncovering of moral dimensions of psychiatric nursing practice); it may be more explicitly didactic (Altschul speaking from her experience to the student or nurse concerned with the main issues facing psychiatric nurses today), or represent a process of care through an intertextual account (Barker and Whitehill).

(5) The contributors address the concern which binds American and British mental health nursing discourses: patient–nurse interaction and the patient–nurse relationship (Tilley, 1995a). In the texts we see the nurse in relation to people in distress who are shunned or sidelined by others, in various situations and circumstances. Questions raised for the contributors include: Why is the person here? What does the person need? What is the person's experience, and what does it mean? What are my obligations to my employer, and what to this person? Some particular aspect of the patient-and-nurse-in-context stands out in each chapter. We note the patient: (i) in relation to the setting (group – Tennant, dyad – Barker and Whitehill, a nursing or social care setting – Watson); (ii) as co-agent (Barker and Whitehill's notion of the patient-and-nurse acting together, agent and agency conflated); (iii) as agency (the patient as the means of economic production, in Glenister); (iv) in the act (Pollock's patients making multiple suicide attempts); (v) as the motive (Altschul – to know the patient, Ritter – to mediate between the patient and the psychiatrist, and between the patient's inner and outer worlds); (vi) as metonymic extension, in Gallop's view of nurses acting to advance their and patients' interests as women, or in Walsh's view of nurses acting to recognise, respect and protect difference of various kinds. The patient is thus the focus, but in different ways, depending on the different 'ratios' of the elements of the narratives: act, actor, means, setting, motive.

(6) Mental health nursing is not static, but evolves historically. The basic dynamic of mental health nursing practice conveyed through the chapters, while recognisably akin to the theme of patient–nurse interaction established by Peplau (1988) and Altschul (1972), is nonetheless different. The patient and nurse in these accounts are less individualised and decontextualised than they were in those earlier works. For example, gender and class, treated as relatively unproblematic analytical variables in Altschul (1972), are examined more fully and critically in the chapters by Gallop and Glenister. And, while all the chapters in this volume can be read as con-

cordant with Peplau's (1988) idea that the person the patient becomes depends on the person the nurse becomes, the ideal of democratic discipline espoused by Peplau is displaced by the image of nursing as situated resistance. Watson resists the optimistic paradigm; Tennant resists psychiatrists' categories and forms of care; Glenister resists institutionalised coercion and control; Tilley resisted, unsuccessfully, the pressure of colleagues; Parkes resists the 'old' ways of psychiatric nursing as she experienced them; Walsh resists ignorance of difference; Gallop resists collusion with male psychiatrists' disregard for the issues of power in care for women with borderline personality disorder; Ryan resists pressure towards surrendering to apparent either/or choice in a situation of chronic tension; Barker and Whitehill resist displacement of the patient or client from the centre of care; Pollock resists a view of management that ignores its vital role in creating the possibilities for care and development of patients and nurses; Altschul resists abandonment of the psychiatric nurse or mental nurse, and of the mentally ill; Ritter describes psychiatric nurses' resistance, both to what they regard as illegitimate psychiatric authority, and to recognising their own participation in structures of authority. To be concerned enough to resist these non-therapeutic or anti-therapeutic forces is to situate oneself in a radical understanding of what nursing is. Mental health nursing is a good, pursuit of which requires appropriate knowledge and nous regarding the workings of power.

Being part of the conversation

I noted in the 'Introduction' that some of the contributors, experienced practitioners and writers, said that they found writing about themselves difficult. From this we can draw two conclusions. The first is that mental health nursing practitioners and educators should not underestimate the demands placed on *students* when asked to demonstrate reflective practice through production of narratives of personal experience. Unless teachers and mentors or preceptors undertake such writing-work themselves, they are unlikely to understand the difficulties entailed. Yet, insofar as practice may be 'designed' to enable or require practitioners to do their work non-reflexively (to 'bumper-swing', as Tennant noted, or to evade critical thinking, as Ritter suggests), such a development by and for teachers and experienced practitioners might shake the foundations of practice.

The second conclusion is more a step into imagination justified by the book's form and content. I have represented the chapters as 'versions' of the nurse, and have referred to the authors' voices 'embodied' in these texts. The 'voices' speak to each other, and against any over-riding authorial voice (including this one). 'Conversation' is therefore an apt metaphor for the book. One contributor recalled having, as a student, read the work of another contributor, and said that she never thought that her work and work by the older woman would be in the same book. When reading another we do not know when we may be writing with them. Another contributor, Ryan, noted that the third part of his analysis of the ambiguities of nursing (in the present volume) emerged 2 years after the earlier parts, marking a new stage in self-recognition. So some writings meet their responses from others or from self only with the passage of time and the readiness of others or self to participate in a new conversation. To write is to interact.

I sent my chapter to my friend of 'episode three'. He liked the way I had brought the three episodes together for this book's audience. However, he noted some differences between his interpretation and my interpretation of the episodes narrated. He said that he had not intended to burden me in the first pub conversation, nor to 'sway' me. He had been looking for what he called 'a sympathetic ear'. He thought that his own telling of his story had been somewhat 'staccato', missing something of the meaning and emotional tone of his experience. He thought, moreover, that my account indicated that I had missed some connections and links in what he had experienced and intended to say. Maybe, he thought, a 'gap' is inevitable, between what is experienced and what is told, what is told and what is heard, what is heard and what is written.

Rather than focus on that 'gap' as the key problem and topic for analysis (as might a post-modernist), my friend emphasised that he sought out and valued those people who might, listening with that sympathetic ear, understand him. Perhaps through such conversations he seeks – we all seek – the smallest gap.

That move from 'my friend' to 'we all' is an act of faith entailing two further enlargements of view. One is to see the conversation between my friend and me as an apt metaphor for the 'conversation' among the contributors to this book, and between them and the book's readers. The second step is to see that the younger contributor's recall of her earlier reading, Ryan's mulling unawares over his incomplete analysis, my return to the three episodes, all imply that we *are* in some sense a series of conversations over time, some held with others and some with ourselves. In the conversations we address both other(s) and ourselves. The function of such conversations might be to narrow, not close, the gaps between other(s) and self (my friend's hope) and among the selves we are. The metaphor can be extended yet further, to suggest that this closing of gaps is a form of 'healing', strengthening through conversation the interconnection within self and between self and other(s) which creates or restores a sense of belonging, fulfils a 'longing to belong' (my friend's phrase).

That the contributors' 'versions' are varied, potentially both in accord *and* incongruent, indicates that, in taking our places in conversations – in the conversation linking each and all conversations – we draw on different frameworks for understanding. These frameworks are in effect matrices, 'place(s) in which (things are) developed' (*The Concise Oxford Dictionary*, 1976). If there is one 'thing' which concerns the contributors here, and I hope the reader, it is the response of self developing over time in conversations with self, patients or clients, and other nurses. Response is here considered voice spoken by *and* speaking being 'in relation to other' in time and place. Because each voice both speaks *and* is spoken by a different being, no single framework or 'theory' or 'model', can sustain the conversations we need.

In constructing their 'versions' of the mental health nurse, the contributors have represented their experience and understandings based on experience. We are 'born into the conversation', but each self, each person, patient and nurse, develops in a matrix of conversation afforded by self and by others.* As Shotter (1993, p. 6) argues, 'our ability as individuals to speak representationally ... arises out of us first and primarily speaking in a way that is responsive to the others around us'. How we construct ourselves depends on who the 'others around us' are, in practice and in readership. When the reader articulates her or his own version of nursing, the voices gathered here will find their true response.

References

Altschul, A. (1972) *Patient–Nurse Interaction*. Churchill Livingstone, Edinburgh.
Barker, P.J. & Reynolds, B. (1996) Rediscovering the proper focus of nursing: a critique of Gournay's position on nursing theory and models. *Journal of Psychiatric and Mental Health Nursing* 3 (1), 76–80.
Barker, P.J., Reynolds, W. & Ward, T. (1995) The proper focus of nursing: a critique of the 'caring ideology'. *International Journal of Nursing Studies* 32 (4), 386–397.
Burke, K. (1969) *A Grammar of Motives*. University of California Press, Berkeley.
Gournay, K. (1995) What to do with nursing models. *Journal of Psychiatric and Mental Health Nursing* 2 (5), 325–327.
Peplau, H. (1988) *Interpersonal Relations in Nursing: A Conceptual Frame of Reference for Psychodynamic Nursing*. MacMillan, Basingstoke.
Reynolds, W. & Cormack, D. (1990) *Psychiatric and Mental Health Nursing: Theory and Practice*. Chapman and Hall, London.
Shotter, J. (1993) *Conversational Realities: Constructing Life Through Language*. Sage, London.
The Concise Oxford Dictionary, 7th edn (1976) Oxford University Press, Oxford.
Tilley, S. (1995a) *Negotiating Realities*. Avebury, Aldershot.
Tilley, S. (1995b) Notes on narrative knowledge in psychiatric nursing. *Journal of Psychiatric and Mental Health Nursing* 2 (2), 217–226.

---

* As emblem of this assertion, I note that I have tried but failed to trace the source of the phrase 'born into the conversation': I may have heard it from, or read it in some work by, Miller Mair or Rom Harré.

Index